German Eugenicists

Contents

Chapter 1

Wolfgang Abel

For other people of the same name, see Wolfgang Abel and Mario Furlan.

Wolfgang Abel (13 May 1905 – 1 November 1997) was an Austrian anthropologist and one of Nazi Germany's racial biologists. He was the son of the Austrian paleontologist Othenio Abel.

From 1931 Wolfgang Abel was engaged at the Kaiser Wilhelm Institute of Anthropology, Human Heredity, and Eugenics. In 1933 he became a member of the NSDAP. He was involved in compulsory sterilization of children, who resulted from relationships between German women and dark-skinned French soldiers. In 1934 he wrote an article, which was published in the German newspaper "*Neues Volk*", with the title "*Bastarde am Rhein*" (Rhineland Bastards). In 1935 he joined the SS. In 1942 Abel was successor to Eugen Fischer for the professorship of racial biology at the University of Berlin.

Wolfgang Abel delivered in 1938 a speech at the "Congres International des Sciences Anthropologiques et Ethnologiques, Deuxieme Session, Copenhague 1938. The topic was: Die Rasse der rumänischen Zigeuner. Meaning, On the Race of the Rumanian Gypsies.

In the same year Abel was in addition to his work at the KWI lecturer in anthropology, as well as Deputy Head of the Department of racial hygiene of the German High School for Politics .After joining the SS in 1935, he worked as an expert for the race and settlement main office (RuSHA) of the SS and as Chief Appraiser for the Imperial Family Office. At the Kaiser Wilhelm Institute, Wolfgang Abel rose in 1940 to the head of Department of Ethnography. In July 1941, he was appointed extraordinary Professor. Previously already Assistant of Eugenics to Eugen Fischer, he was from 1943 to 1945 his successor to the Chair of professorship in the University of Berlin. At the same time, he worked at this time for the high command of the German Army (OKH). In the framework of the General Plan East, Abel worked out a plan for a "progressive elimination" of the "Russian race' with which he wanted all "Russian Nordic types "Germanized" and the rest deported to Siberia, in May 1942.

In addition to his teaching Wolfgang Abel assumed the management of the Institute Awards of the German High School for Politics in 1943. In 1945, Abel was dismissed from the University of Berlin. From 1945 to 1947 he was interned. He then lived as a portrait painter in Austria.

After World War II, he lived in Austria until his death in 1997.

1.1 References

1.2 Literature

- Ernst Klee ("Das Personenlexikon zum Dritten Reich") describes Wolfgang Abel as an anthropologist who joined the NSDAP in 1933 and in 1935 joined the SS, was attached to SS-RuSHA and was Leiter des Institutes für Rassenbiologie der Deutschen Hochschule für Politik. Klee gives him a birthdate of 13.05.1905.

- Lusane, Clarence (2002). *Hitler's Black Victims: The Historical Experience of Afro-Germans, European Blacks, Africans and African Americans in the Nazi Era (Cross Currents in African American History)* Routledge. ISBN 978-0-415-93295-0

- Proctor, Robert (2006). *Racial Hygiene: Medicine Under the Nazis* Harvard University Press. ISBN 978-0-674-74578-0

Chapter 2

Otto Ammon

Otto Georg Ammon (December 7, 1842 in Karlsruhe, Baden – January 14, 1916 in Karlsruhe) was a German anthropologist. Ammon was an engineer from 1863 to 1868. In 1883 he led a geographical and geological exploration of Roman roads. In 1887 he conducted anthropological research and from 1887 onwards he was a member of the Ancient Karlsruher Association and the Natural Science Association. In 1904 he received an honorary doctorate from the University of Freiburg.

He is best known for his masterwork, "Natural Selection among Humans" (1883), in which he argued that a significantly higher proportion of persons of Germanic ancestry are to be found within the European aristocracies.

2.1   Literary works

- *Natürliche Auslese beim Menschen*, 1893 (Natural selection among humans)

- *Zur Anthropologie der Badener*, 1899 (On the anthropology of the people of Baden)

- *Gesellschaftsordnung und ihre natürliche Anlage*, 1900 (Social order and its natural application)

Chapter 3

Gertrud Bäumer

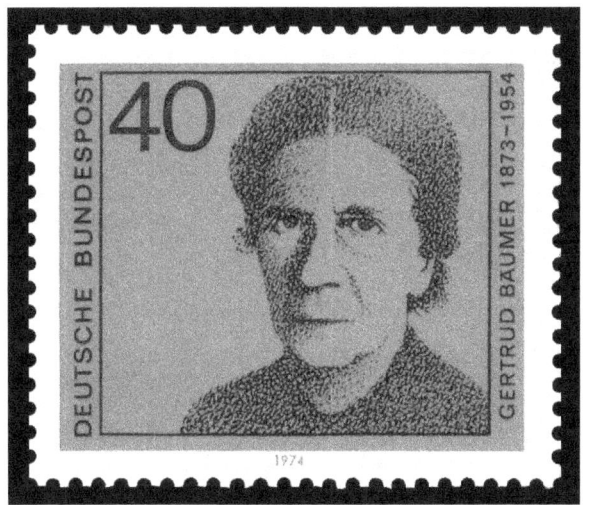

Gertrud Bäumer, German commemorative postage stamp 1974

Gertrud Bäumer (12 September 1873, Hagen-Hohenlimburg, Westphalia – 25 March 1954, Bethel) was a German politician who actively participated in the German civil rights feminist movement. She was also a writer, and contributed to Friedrich Naumann's paper *Die Hilfe*. From 1898, Bäumer lived and worked together with the German feminist and politician Helene Lange.[1]

3.1 Life

Bäumer was a member in close contact with the board of the national umbrella group of German women's organizations, the *Bund Deutscher Frauenvereine* (Federation of German Women's Associations), and during World War I supported the *Nationaler Frauendienst* (National Women's Service). As such, Bäumer was aggressively opposed to the feminist-pacifist women supporting internationalism in Germany and elsewhere; stating: "We mustn't ever forget that it is not just military training that is being put to the test out there in the trenches and at sea, at the gun emplacements and in the air, but also German mothers' upbringing and German wives' care."[2] After the war she joined the German Democratic Party, for which she was a Reichstag member between 1919 and 1932.

3.2 References

[1] "Helene Lange 1848-1930; Frauenrechtlerin, Politikerin (in English: Helene Lange 1848-1930; Women's Rights Activist, Politician)". *Lebendiges Museum Online*. Deutsches Historisches Museum, Berlin. Retrieved 24 June 2015.

[2] G. Bäumer (1914) 'Der Krieg und die Frau', in E. Jäckh (ed.) *Der deutsche Krieg: Politische Flugschriften* (Stuttgart: Deutsche Verlagsanstalt), p. 11.

3.3 Further reading

- Schaser, Angelika (2000). *Helene Lange und Gertrud Bäumer: eine politische Lebensgemeinschaft* [*Helene Lange and Gertrud Bäumer: a political cohabitation*] (in German). Köln Weimar: Böhlau Verlag. ISBN 9783412091002.

- Repp, K. (2000). "⍰�More Corporeal, More Concrete": Liberal Humanism, Eugenics, and German Progressives at the Last Fin de Siècle*". *The Journal of Modern History* **72** (3): 683–730. doi:10.1086/316045. replacement character in |title= at position 2 (help)

- Repp, Kevin (2000). *Reformers, Critics, and the Paths of German Modernity*. Cambridge: Harvard University Press. ISBN 0-674-00057-9.

3.4 External links

- (German) Biographie: Gertrud Bäumer, 1873-1954 at the *Deutsches Historisches Museum*

- Online Biography of Gertrud Bäumer (in German)

Chapter 4

Karl Binding

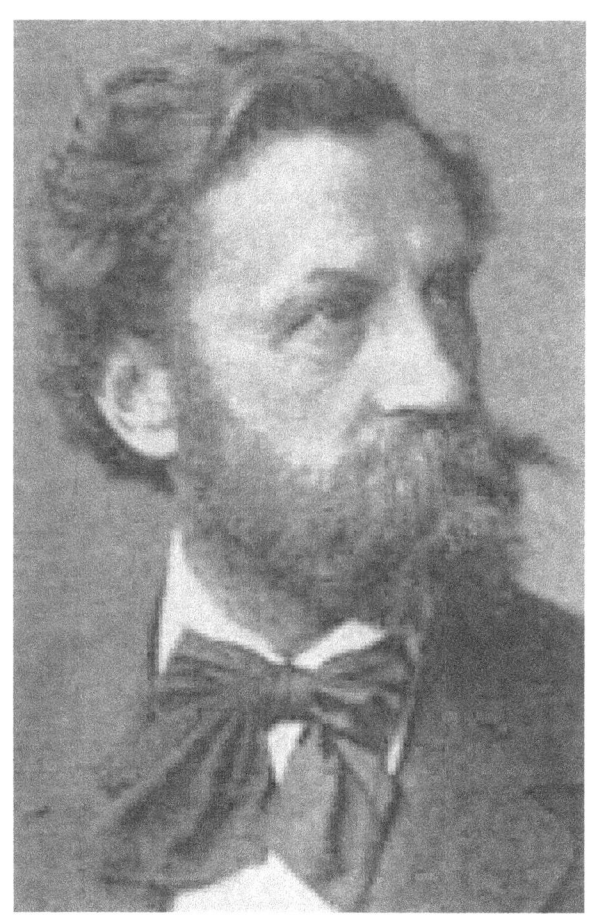

Karl Binding

Karl Ludwig Lorenz Binding (June 4, 1841 – April 7, 1920) was a German jurist known as a promoter of the theory of retributive justice. His influential book, *Die Freigabe der Vernichtung lebensunwerten Lebens* ("Allowing the Destruction of Life Unworthy of Living"), written together with the psychiatrist Alfred Hoche, was used by the Nazis to justify their T-4 Euthanasia Program.[1]

4.1 Life

Binding was born in Frankfurt am Main, the third child of Georg Christoph Binding and Dorothea Binding.

In 1860 Binding moved to Göttingen where he studied history and jurisprudence. After a short stay in Heidelberg, where he won a law prize, he moved back to Göttingen to finish his studies. In 1864 he completed his *habilitation* paper in Latin about Roman criminal law and lectured in criminal law at Heidelberg University. Two years later he was appointed professor of law of state and criminal law and procedure in Basel, Switzerland. In the same year he married Marie Luise Wirsing and published *Das burgundisch-romanische Königreich* and *Entwurf eines Strafgesetzbuches für den Norddeutschen Bund*. At this time he also became friends with Johann Jacob Bernoulli - an archaeologist, Jakob Burckhardt - an art historian, and Friedrich Nietzsche - a philosopher. In August 1867 his first son, Rudolf Georg, was born, followed two years later by his second son. Rudolf G Binding later became a famous writer. Karl Binding and his wife were to have one more son and two daughters. In 1869 his family moved to Freiburg, and Binding volunteered to fight in the Franco-Prussian War. Although his lack of military training meant he was unable to serve as a soldier, he was accepted as an orderly and posted to the front, serving in a field hospital. In 1872 he took on a post at the Reichs University in Straßburg. In the same year he moved to Leipzig University, where he was to continue to work for the next 40 years. From 1879 until to 1900 Binding worked in the district court of Leipzig. After becoming Leipzig University's rector and receiving his emeritus, he moved to Freiburg, where his wife died only a few days later at 71 years old. In 1918, during the First World War, Binding left Germany to lecture German soldiers in Macedonia and Bulgarian intellectuals in Sofia.

4.2 Ideas

4.2.1 Allowing the destruction of life unworthy of living: *Die Freigabe der Vernichtung Lebensunwerten Lebens*

This was the title of one of Binding's most infamous books, co-written by the psychiatrist, Alfred Hoche.[2] The book was divided into two parts, the first written by Binding, the second by Hoche. Binding discussed the consequences that the legal status of suicide would have on euthanasia and the legality of killing the mentally ill. Hoche concentrated on the relationship of doctors to their patients and the seriously ill. (See Alfred Hoche.) Binding and Hoche are noted for the influence their work had on the Nazis and especially the Aktion T4 Euthanasia Program.

4.2.2 Two possible interpretations of German law

In Binding's own interpretation of the law in 1920s Germany, suicide or attempting suicide was not illegal and should be treated as being within the law. This would mean that no-one would have the right to stop a person from killing themselves and that a person who wants to die would not even have the right to defend themselves against such an attempt.

Binding goes on to assume that the right to suicide would then also have to be transferable to another person; meaning that a person also has the right to let someone else cause their death if they so wish. In this case, anyone that has killed a seriously ill person, acting on the behalf of that person, has acted within the law.

Binding's second possible interpretation of German law meant that suicide was neither legal nor illegal. He argued that the law concerning murder only referred to the killing of other people and not to suicide. In this case suicide would be perfectly legal, but euthanasia, involving the killing of another person, even with their permission would have to be treated as murder.

Again if suicide is not illegal, then no-one can stop another person from killing themselves. Binding noted that in reality, the majority of people who prevent a suicide attempt are not usually prosecuted and that most people who are prevented from killing themselves do not make a second attempt. He was of the opinion that in a case of prosecution due to euthanasia, the court should differentiate between the taking of a healthy life and a terminally ill person.

4.2.3 Definition of euthanasia

Binding defined euthanasia as occurring when a person gives a terminally ill person, with the intention of reducing pain, a medicine which either immediately or eventually leads to that person's painless death.

For a case of euthanasia to stay within the law, the medicine must enable the person to die painlessly at or around the same time as they would have otherwise died. In this way the doctor is simply exchanging the cause of death, from a painful one caused by illness to a painless one caused by a medicament. Any killing which involves the shortening of a life was seen as unlawful.

Binding claimed the killing of the terminally ill was not an exception to the law against murder but was a lawful act in the interests of the patient. It put an end to their terrible suffering and should not be seen as a killing but as a reduction in their suffering. Binding did not think it necessary to obtain permission from a person who was to be killed, but if they were able to and expressed the wish to live, that wish must be respected.

Binding split the group of people which he wanted to be considered for killing into three groups, "two larger ones and a middle group".

- 1 A person who has been mortally wounded or is terminally ill and has somehow communicated their wish to die.

The person does not have to be in pain, it is enough that they are in a helpless condition and that their condition is incurable. It is also irrelevant if the person could be saved in another situation.

- 2 A person that is incurably mentally ill.

Binding describes these people as having neither the will to die, nor the will to live. They are "living pointless lives and are a burden for society and their families". He also believed it to be unfair on carers to keep such "lives unworthy of living" alive.

- 3 The people belonging to the middle group, were "mentally healthy" people, which having suffered a serious injury are now unconscious. If they ever awake, they "will awake to a nameless suffering".

"Their killing should not be seen as a killing as such but as saving the person from a terrible end."

Binding could not work out a general rule for the killing of this group. Importantly he accepted that many killings of these people would actually be unjustifiable, although this would only be evident after death. He believed that the law would treat such killings as manslaughter. This led him to argue for a new law to allow for such killings which according with his views would have been "justifiable".

Binding wanted a committee to decide on a killing on a case by case basis. The committee was to consist of a doctor, a psychiatrist or other doctor and a jurist to check that the committee was acting within the law. The committee would be able to call witnesses and was also to have a chairperson - without voting rights - to run the proceedings. Neither the applicant nor their doctor could be members of the committee. An applicant could represent themselves, be represented by their doctor, family or anyone they had asked. Binding was of the opinion "that it is quite possible for a person under the age of 18 or for the mentally ill" to decide whether they want to live or die.

After a committee had checked that a person fulfils the criteria, it could make a decision. For a decision to be final, it would have to be agreed upon by all three parties and must be made purely out of pity and the killing must be done painlessly. Any person could withdraw their application to be killed at any time, including after the decision had been finalised. In the case of an unconscious person or the mentally ill, Binding allowed the final decision to be made by the mother. If the family were willing to take on the person themselves or pay the costs of hospitalisation, the person would not be killed. In the case of a conscious person the person's wishes were to be respected regardless of the interests or requests of the family.

4.2.4 Killings without the jurisdiction of a committee

Binding also wanted to allow for killings that were not controlled by a committee. Such a killing would only be legal if the person killing had either acted with permission, or on the assumption that an unconscious person wanted to die. After the death a committee must be able to be satisfied that the killing fulfilled all of the usual requirements.

Binding argued that although there is always a possibility of killing the wrong person, "that which is good and reasonable must take place irrespective of any possibility of error". He saw the risk of losing a life as unimportant because "humanity constantly loses so many lives by mistake, that just one more would hardly make a difference".

4.3 Publications by Binding

- Das burgundisch-romanische Königreich: Geschichte des burgundisch-romanischen Königreichs
- Entwurf eines Strafgesetzbuches für den Norddeutschen Bund
- Die Normen und ihre Übertretung. Eine Untersuchung über die rechtmäßige Handlung und die Arten des Delikts
- Die Freigabe der Vernichtung lebensunwerten Lebens, Hoche A, Binding, K. Felix Meiner Verlag, Leipzig, 1920 (2nd Edition 1922)

4.4 Publications about Binding

- Kaufmann, Arnim: Lebendiges und Totes in Bindings Normentheorie, Schwartz 1954
- Klaus-Peter Drechsel: Beurteilt Vermessen Ermordet. Praxis der Euthanasie bis zum Ende des deutschen Faschismus. Duisburg 1993, ISBN 3-927388-37-8
- Ernst Klee, «Euthanasie» im NS-Staat. Die «Vernichtung lebensunwerten Lebens», Fischer Taschenbuch Verlag, Frankfurt a.M. 1985
- Rezension mit dem Titel „Vernichtung lebensunwerten Lebens", verfaßt von Dr.F. Limacher aus Bern, Internationales Ärztliches Bulletin, Dezember 1934, Nummer 12 (Erscheinungsort: Prag), 181-183, hier 183, neu erschienen in Beiträge zur nationalsozialistischen Gesundheits- und Sozialpolitik, Band 7, Internationales Ärztliches Bulletin, Jahrgang I-VI (1934-1939), Reprint, Rotbuch Verlag, Berlin 1989.

4.5 See also

- Eugen Fischer

4.6 References

[1] Henry Friedlander (1997). *The Origins of Nazi Genocide: From Euthanasia to the Final Solution.*

[2] https://de.wikipedia.org/w/index.php?title=Datei: BindingHoche_FreigabeCoverAufl22.jpg

4.7 External links

- Works by Karl Binding at Project Gutenberg
- Works by or about Karl Binding at Internet Archive
- Allowing the Destruction of Life Unworthy of Life - English translation
- Die Freigabe der Vernichtung lebensunwerten Lebens - Original version

Chapter 5

Agnes Bluhm

Agnes Bluhm (9 January 1862 – 12 November 1943) was a German winner of a Goethe medal. She was trained as a medical doctor and won prizes for her research. She believed that German women could improve the race using eugenics and forced sterilisation. She wrote that the "female psyche" made her gender predisposed towards working for "racial hygiene".

5.1   Life

Bluhm was born in Constantinople in 1862. She was trained as a medical doctor and won prizes for her research. She believed that German women could improve the race using eugenics.[1]

In 1886 she fell in love with Alfred Ploetz who was already involved with another scientist named Pauline Rüdin. They became involved whilst conducting dissection and they decided to get married early in 1887. Ploetz was also seeing an American named Mary Sherwood who was studying hypnotism. Ploetz returned to Rudin in 1888 and married her. Bluhm however kept Ploetz as a close friend throughout her life and they both shared similar views on racial purity and the benefits of eugenics.[2]

Bluhm became the third female doctor in Berlin and she joined two fellow Zurich trained doctors to staff a clinic for poor women there in 1890.[3] She joined the Racial Hygiene Society in 1906.[2]

Bluhm had to retire from practising medicine due to problems with her ears but she redirected her efforts to medical research. After 1918 she conducted extensive research on heredity in animals to try and determine how a race could be improved.[1] She is said to be first German female doctor known for her research.[3] She carried out research on Alcoholism and Heredity under early funding from the Rockefeller Foundation. Bluhm was awarded a silver Leibnitz medal for her work.[1]

In 1936 she published her book which laid out her views on the role of women. *The Racial Hygiene Problem for Women Physicians* described how she saw women's role to work hard at reproduction in order to improve humanity. Women should look to motherhood and not to emancipation as their contribution. Although Bluhm had a career she saw this as a special case because of the need for speciality doctors. In general she thought that women should not have careers. Moreover she recommended that the "female psyche" made her gender predisposed towards working for "racial hygiene".[1]

She won the Goethe-Medaille für Kunst und Wissenschaft during the war. Adolf Hitler awarded about 400 of these medals during his time in power but only five were awarded to women and the rest were a singer, actresses and writers.[4]

Bluhm died in Beelitz in 1943 before the end of the Second World War (Some say 1944[1]).

5.2   References

[1] Ogilvie t al, Marilyn (2000). *Biographical Dictionary of Women in Science*. pp. 305–307. ISBN 1135963436.

[2] Weindling, Paul (1993). *Health, race, and German politics between national unification and Nazism, 1870-1945* (1st pbk. ed.). Cambridge: Cambridge University Press. p. 74. ISBN 052142397X.

[3] Creese, Mary R. S. Creese ; with contributions by Thomas M. (2004). *West European women in science, 1800 - 1900 : a survey of their contributions to research*. Lanham, Md. [u.a.]: Scarecrow Press. p. 160. ISBN 0810849798.

[4] Heyck, Hartmut. *The Goethe-Medal for Art and Science*. lulu.com. p. 26. ISBN 0981218202.

Chapter 6

Hermann Boehm (eugenicist)

For other people of the same name, see Hermann Böhm.

Hermann Alois Boehm (27 October 1884, Fürth,

1&text=nur_13tr

6.2 Bibliography

- R.Procor, *Racial hygiene - medicine under the Nazis*, (Cambridge, Mass., Harvard University Press, 1988)

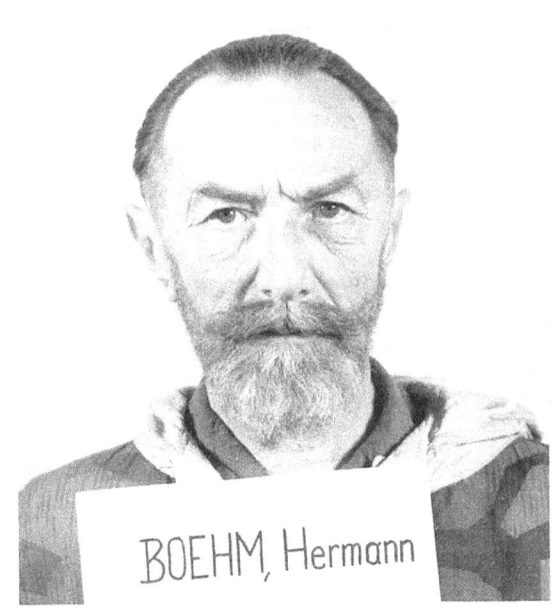

Hermann Boehm at the Nuremberg Trials (1947)

Bavaria - 7 June 1962, Gießen) was a German eugenicist, doctor, professor of 'Racial Hygiene' and SA-Sanitäts-Gruppenführer during the National Socialist era. Hermann Boehm became a member of the Nazi party on March 24, 1925 with registration number 120. Boehm was an ordinary professor of racial improvement at Giessen from January 1, 1943 until the end of World War II.[1]

6.1 Notes

[1] http://nuremberg.law.harvard.edu/php/docs_swi.php?DI=

Chapter 7

Werner Catel

Werner Catel (27 June 1894 – 30 April 1981), Professor of Neurology and Psychiatry at the University of Leipzig, was one of three doctors considered an expert on the programme of euthanasia for children and participated in the Action T4 "euthanasia" program for the Nazis, the other two being Hans Heinze and Ernst Wentzler.

In early 1939 a farm labourer called Richard Kretschmar requested Catel's permission to euthanize one of his children, now identified as Gerhard Kretschmar, who had been born blind and deformed. Catel deferred the matter and suggested the father write directly to Hitler for permission. Hitler subsequently sent Dr. Karl Brandt to confer with Catel and decide on a course of action. On July 25, 1939 the child was killed.

The T4 program was influenced by a popular book written in 1920 by Alfred Hoche and Karl Binding. Catel as part of this program was surely influenced by it, too. In his 1962 publication, *"Grenzsituation des Lebens"* (Border situations of life), Catel argued for the reintroduction of euthanasia. As had Binding and Hoche, Catel identified three possible types of euthanasia.

- *Reine Euthanasie*:

"Real" euthanasia was seen as the killing of a person who was suffering from so much pain, that an ever increasing amount of pain reducing drugs had to be administered. This consequently lead to the person's death.

- *Euthanasie im engeren Sinne*:

The killing of a patient whose illness "according to medical experience" is so bad "that there is no hope of recovery", but whose death is also not to be expected in the near future. (See terminal sedation)

- *Euthanasie im weiteren Sinne*:

The "extermination of the life of an "idiot child" or an adult in a similar condition. Catel defined "idiot children" as

being "such monsters ... which are nothing but a massa carnis"(Martin Luther), have no personality or spiritual soul (Guardini), are unable to make decisions (Thomas More) or are unable to communicate with their surroundings.(Alfred Hoche)

After the war Catel took charge of the *Mammolshöhe Children's Mental Home* near Kronberg, where he continued to rally for the euthanasia of children deemed beyond hope. In 1949 he was found to have committed no grave crimes by a denazification board in Hamburg, and became attached to the University of Kiel in 1954. There was talk after his death in 1981, of establishing a *Werner Catel Foundation* with $200,000 of unclaimed money left after his death, but the idea was finally dismissed in 1984.

7.1 See also

- Alfred Hoche

- Karl Binding

- Life unworthy of life

7.2 Trivia

- Catel was the first physician to describe what is now known as Lesch-Nyhan syndrome

- His obituary controversially stated that he acted "in many ways, to the welfare and well-being of sick children."

7.3 References

- Hans-Christian Petersen und Sönke Zankel. *Werner Catel - ein Protagonist der NS-"Kindereuthanasie" und seine Nachkriegskarriere*. In: Medizinhistorisches

Journal. Medicine and the Life Sciences in History 38 (2003), S. 139-173.

- Hans-Christian Petersen und Sönke Zankel: *"Ein exzellenter Kinderarzt, wenn man von den Euthanasie-Dingen einmal absieht." - Werner Catel und die Vergangenheitspolitik der Universität Kiel.* In: Hans-Werner Prahl u. a. (Hrsg.): Uni-Formierung des Geistes. Universität Kiel und der Nationalsozialismus. Kiel 2007, Bd. 2, S. 133-179.

- Ernst Klee: *Deutsche Medizin im Dritten Reich*, S. Fischer Verlag Frankfurt/M., Oktober 2001 (Besprechung auf graswurzel.net)

- Manfred Müller-Küppers: *Die Geschichte der Kinder- und Jugendpsychiatrie unter besonderer Berücksichtigung der Zeit des Nationalsozialismus* kinderpsychiater.org

- Ortrun Riha: *Das schwerbehinderte Kind als ethische Verantwortung. Die Bürde der Vergangenheit als Verantwortung für die Zukunft.* In: *110 Jahre Universitätsklinik und Poliklinik für Kinder und Jugendliche in Leipzig.* Basel 2003, S. 17 ff.

- Joachim Karl Dittrich: *Rechtfertigungen? Betrachtungen zu drei Buchveröffentlichungen Werner Catels.* In: 110 Jahre Universitätsklinik und Poliklinik für Kinder und Jugendliche in Leipzig. Basel 2003, S. 27 ff.

- Berit Lahm, Thomas Seyde, Eberhard Ulm: *Kindereuthanasieverbrechen in Leipzig. Verantwortung und Rezeption.* Plöttner Verlag, Leipzig 2008, ISBN 978-3-938442-48-7.

7.4 External links

- Books by and about Catel in the German National Bibliography

- Page on Catel in the Faculty Catalog of the University of Leipzig

- Beitrag von Udo Benzenhöfer Article by Udo Benzenhöfer (PDF, 162 kB) In: German Medical Journal, Vol 97, Issue 42, October 20, 2000

- interview with Catel in *Der Spiegel,* 19.02.1964

*srticle on Catel in *Der Spiegel* 8/24/1960

Chapter 8

Eugen Fischer

For the historian, see Eugen Fischer (historian).

Eugen Fischer (5 July 1874 – 9 July 1967) was a German professor of medicine, anthropology and eugenics. He was director of the Kaiser Wilhelm Institute of Anthropology, Human Heredity, and Eugenics between 1927 and 1942. He was appointed rector of the Frederick William University of Berlin by Adolf Hitler in 1933, and later joined the Nazi Party.

8.1 Biography

Fischer was born in Karlsruhe, Grand Duchy of Baden, in 1874. Fischer studied medicine, folkloristics and history from 1893–1898 in Berlin, Freiburg and Munich. Promotion to Dr. med in 1898 and in 1900 habilitation for anatomy and anthropology at the University of Freiburg.[1] He became Director of the Anatomical Institute in Freiburg in 1918,[2] part of the University of Freiburg.[3]

In 1927, Fischer became the director of the Kaiser Wilhelm Institute of Anthropology, Human Heredity, and Eugenics (KWI-A), a role for which he'd been recommended the prior year by Erwin Baur.[4]

In 1933 Fischer signed the *Loyalty Oath of German Professors to Adolf Hitler and the National Socialist State*.

In 1933, Adolf Hitler appointed him rector of the Frederick William University of Berlin, now Humboldt University.[5] Fischer retired from the university in 1942.

Otmar Freiherr von Verschuer was a student of Fischer, Verschuer himself had a prominent pupil, Josef Mengele.[6][7]

After the war, he completed his memoirs, which critics claim whitewash his role in the genocidal program of the Third Reich. He died in 1967.

8.2 Early work

In 1908 Fischer conducted field research in German Southwest Africa (now Namibia). He studied the Basters, offspring of German or Boer men who had fathered children by the native women (Hottentots) in that area. His study concluded with a call to prevent a "mixed race" by the prohibition of "mixed marriage" such as those he had studied. It included unethical medical practices on the Herero and Namaqua people.[8] He argued that while the existing Mischling descendants of the mixed marriages might be useful for Germany, he recommended that they should not continue to reproduce. His recommendations were followed and by 1912 interracial marriage was prohibited throughout the German colonies.[9][10] As a precursor to his experiments on Jews in Nazi Germany, he collected bones and skulls for his studies, in part from medical experimentation on African prisoners of war in Namibia during the Herero and Namaqua Genocide.[11][12]

His ideas expressed in this work, related to maintaining the purity of races, influenced future German legislation on race, including the Nuremberg laws.[10]

8.3 Nazi Germany

In the years of 1937–1938 Fischer and his colleagues analysed 600 children in Nazi Germany descending from French-African soldiers who occupied western areas of Germany after First World War; the children were subsequently subjected to sterilization afterwards.[13]

Fischer didn't officially join the Nazi Party until 1940.[14] However, he was influential with National Socialists early on. A two-volume work, *Foundations of Human Hereditary Teaching and Racial Hygiene* published 1921 and 1932, and in 1936 published under *Human Heredity Theory and Racial Hygiene*, co-written by Erwin Baur and Fritz Lenz. The book served as the scientific basis for the Nazis' eugenic policies.[15] He also authored *The Rehoboth Bas-*

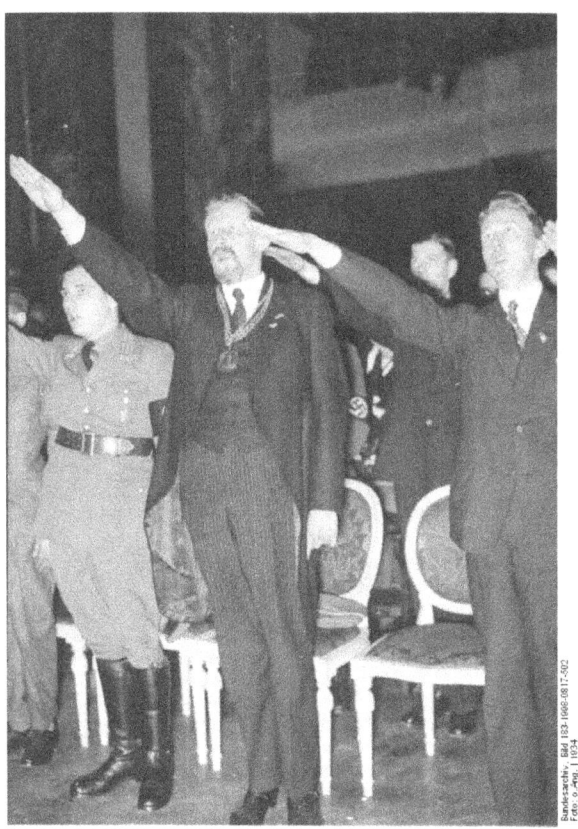

Eugen Fischer during a ceremony at the University of Berlin 1934

tards and the Problem of Miscegenation among Humans (1913) (German: *Die Rehobother Bastards und das Bastardierungsproblem beim Menschen*), a field study which provided context for later racial debates, influenced German colonial legislation and provided scientific support for the Nuremberg laws.[16]

Under the Nazi regime, Fischer developed the physiological specifications used to determine racial origins and developed the so-called Fischer–Saller scale. He and his team experimented on Gypsies and African-Germans, taking blood and measuring skulls to find scientific validation for his theories.

Efforts to return the Namibian skulls taken by Fischer were started with an investigation by the University of Freiburg in 2011 and completed with the return of the skulls in March 2014.[17][18][19]

8.4 Works

8.4.1 To 1909

- Fischer, Eugen. 1899. "Beiträge zur Kenntniss der Nasenhöhle und des Thränennasenganges der Am-

phisbaeniden", *Archiv für Mikroskopische Anatomie*. 55:1, pp. 441–478.

- Fischer, Eugen. 1901. "Zur Kenntniss der Fontanella metopica und ihrer Bildungen". *Zeitschrift für Morphologie und Anthropologie*.4:1. pp. 17–30.

- Fischer, Eugen, Professor an der Universität Freiburg i. Br. 1906. "Die Variationen an Radius und Ulna des Menschen". *Zeitschrift für Morphologie und Anthropologie*. Vol. 9. No. 2.

- Fischer, Eugen. 1908. *Der Patriziat Heinrichs III und Heinrichs IV*. Tübingen: J.C.B. Mohr (Paul Siebeck). Fischer's PhD thesis.

8.4.2 1910 to 1919

- Maass, Alfred. *Durch Zentral-Sumatra*. Berlin: Behr. 1910. Additional contributing authors: J.P. Kleiweg de Zwaan and E. Fischer.

- Fischer, Eugen. 1913.*Die Rehobother Bastards und das Bastardierungsproblem beim Menschen: anthropologische und ethnographiesche Studien am Rehobother Bastardvolk in Deutsch-Südwest-Afrika*, ausgeführt mit Unterstützung der Kgl. preuss, Akademie der Wissenschaften. Jena: G. Fischer.

- Gaupp, Ernst Wilhelm Theodor. Eugen Fischer (ed.) 1917. *August Weismann: sein Leben und sein Werk*. Jena: Verlag von Gustav Fischer.

8.4.3 1920 to 1929

- Schwalbe, G. and Eugen Fischer (eds.). *Anthropologie*. Leipzig: B.G. Teubner, 1923.

- Fischer, E. and H.F.K. Günther. *Deutsche Köpfe nordischer Rasse: 50 Abbildungen mit Geleitwarten*. Munich: J.F. Lehmann. 1927.

8.4.4 1940 to 1949

- Fischer, Eugen and Gerhard Kittel. *Das antike Weltjudentum : Tatsachen, Texte, Bilder*. Hamburg: Hanseatische Verlagsanstalt, 1943.[20]

8.4.5 1950 to 1959

- Sarkar, Sasanka Sekher; Eugen Fischer and Keith Arthur, *The Aboriginal Races of India*, Calcutta: Bookland. 1954.

- Fischer, Eugen. *Begegnungen mit Toten: aus den Erinnerungen eines Anatomen.* Freiburg: H.F. Schulz. 1959.

8.5 See also

- Ex-Nazi
- Karl Binding
- Nazi eugenics
- Racial policies of the Third Reich
- Scientific racism
- Subsequent Nuremberg Trials
- Doctors' Trial
- Anthropometry
- Fischer scale
- Fischer-Saller scale
- Shark Island Concentration Camp

8.6 Notes

[1] Max-Planck-Gesellschaft - Archive. "Fischer, Eugen".

[2] "Eugen Fischer".

[3] Eugen Fischer (1921). "Bitte des anatomischen Instituts Freiburg i.B.".

[4] Schmul 2003, p. 25.

[5] Historische Komission München

[6] Michael H. Kater (2011). "The Nazi Symbiosis: Human Genetics and Politics in the Third Reich". *Bulletin of the History of Medicine* **85**: 515–516. doi:10.1353/bhm.2011.0067.

[7] Randall Hansen, Desmond King (2013). *Sterilized by the State: Eugenics, Race, and the Population Scare in Twentieth-Century.* Cambridge University Press. p. 158. ISBN 1107434599.

[8] http://www.ezakwantu.com/Gallery%20Herero%20and%20Namaqua%20Genocide.htm

[9] *Holocaust Encyclopedia*, p. 420

[10] Friedlander 1997, p. 11

[11] http://www.ezakwantu.com/Gallery%20Herero%20and%20Namaqua%20Genocide.htmMedical experimentation in Africa

[12] Lusane, Clarence (2002-12-13). "Hitler's black victims: The historical experiences of Afro-Germans, European Blacks, Africans, and African Americans in the Nazi era". ISBN 9780415932950.

[13] Bioethics: an anthology Helga Kuhse,Peter Singer page 232 Wiley-Blackwell 2006

[14] "Human biodiversity: genes, race, and history", Jonathan M. Marks. Transaction Publishers, 1995. p. 88. ISBN 0202020339, 9780202020334.

[15] A. E. Samaan (2013). *From a Race of Masters to a Master Race: 1948 To 1848.* A.E. Samaan. p. 539. ISBN 1626600007.

[16] *Holocaust Encyclopedia* p. 420.

[17] "Repatriation of Skulls from Namibia University of Freiburg hands over human remains in ceremony". 2014.

[18] https://www.youtube.com/watch?v=5c-wJDUW89A

[19] http://www.newera.com.na/2014/02/28/germany-send-35-skulls/

[20] *Das Antike Weltjudentum - Forschungen zur Judenfrage.* 1944.

8.7 References

- Baumel, Judith Tydor (2001). *The Holocaust Encyclopedia.* Yale University Press. ISBN 0-300-08432-3.

- Black, Edwin (2004). *War Against the Weak: Eugenics and America's Campaign to Create a Master Race.* Thunder's Mouth Press. ISBN 1-56858-321-4.

- Fangerau H., Müller I. (2002). "Das Standardwerk der Rassenhygiene von Erwin Baur, Eugen Fischer und Fritz Lenz im Urteil der Psychiatrie und Neurologie 1921-1940". *Der Nervenarzt* **73** (11): 1039–1046. doi:10.1007/s00115-002-1421-1. PMID 12430045.

- Mendes-Flohr, Paul R. (1995). *The Jew in the Modern World: A Documentary History.* Oxford University Press US. ISBN 0-19-507453-X.

- Schmuhl, Hans-Walter. "The Kaiser Wilhelm Institute for Anthropology, Human heredity and Eugenics, 1927-1945", Boston Studies in the Philosophy of Science vol. 259, Wallstein Verlag, Göttingen, 2003

- Weindling P. (1985). "Weimar eugenics: The kaiser wilhelm institute for anthropology, human heredity and eugenics in social context". *Annals of Science* **42** (3): 303–318. doi:10.1080/00033798500200221. PMID 11620696.

- Friedlander, Henry. 1997. *The origins of Nazi genocide: from euthanasia to the Final Solution.* University of North Carolina Press. ISBN 0-8078-2208-6 ISBN 0807846759.

8.8 External links

- Book Review of *The Rehoboth Bastards* in *Nature* (1913)

- 2004 Newspaper Article regarding *The Rehoboth Bastards*

- *The Rehoboth Bastards* (Photo Album)

- Herero and Namaqua Genocide - Galerie Ezakwantu

- Lusane, Clarence (2002-12-13). "Hitler's black victims: The historical experiences of Afro-Germans, European Blacks, Africans, and African Americans in the Nazi era". ISBN 978-0-415-93295-0.

- Detailed overview of Eugen Fischer with references

Chapter 9

Hermann Gauch

Hermann Gauch (6 May 1899 – 7 November 1978) was a Nazi race theorist noted for his dedication to Nordic theory to an extent that embarrassed the Nazi leadership when he claimed that Italians were "half ape". Briefly adjutant to Heinrich Himmler, his career was later stalled by Himmler himself. During World War II he served with distinction in the Yugoslav campaign.

After the war he remained devoted to Nazi ideology and Holocaust denial, claiming that Jewish deaths in the Holocaust were exaggerated and becoming an activist in the neo-Nazi Deutsche Reichspartei.[1] His life and ideas were recorded by his politically unsympathetic son Sigfrid Gauch in a memoir which was the first significant example of the genre of "father memoirs" written by the children of former Nazis.

9.1 Early life

Gauch was born in Einöllen. His father was a farmer, who died of malaria in Africa when Hermann was 14. From 1913 to 1917 he studied at Kaiserlautern and Augsburg. In 1917 he joined the German army, participating in the late stages of World War I. He was badly injured at the Battle of Soissons in 1918 and captured by American troops. He escaped from a French prison camp in 1919.[2]

In the post-war years Gauch trained to become a physician, qualifying in 1924. In 1922 he joined the Nazi party, becoming a member of Rudolf Hess's S.A. unit. In 1924 he participated in the assassination of Franz Josef Heinz, leader of the separatist government of the Palatinate. At this time Gauch was closest to the circles of the Nordicist and neopagan faction within the party led by Himmler, Alfred Rosenberg and Walter Darré.[2]

After the Nazi party was disbanded following the Beer Hall Putsch, Gauch's party membership lapsed. He did not renew it in 1925 when the party was re-established because by that time he was employed as a doctor in the Handelsmarine (merchant marine) and later the Kriegsmarine, which pre-

cluded party membership. He rejoined the party in 1934, also becoming a member of the SS. He was briefly Himmler's adjutant for cultural and racial affairs, but was not a success in the post. He resigned from the SS in 1935 after marriage became a requirement for membership. His application to rejoin in 1937 was turned down by Himmler personally.[2]

9.2 Theories

Gauch remained close to Darré, whose vision of the agricultural self-sufficiency of Nordic peasantry he shared. He wrote six books of "race research" while a member of the SS, expressing both antisemitic and Nordicist ideas, emphasising them to an extent that was extreme even in Nazi Germany. He insisted in 1933 that the fact that "birds can be taught to talk better than other animals is explained by the fact that their mouths are Nordic in structure." He further claimed that in humans, "the shape of the Nordic gum allows a superior movement of the tongue, which is the reason why Nordic talking and singing are richer."[3] In 1934 his most important book *New Foundations for Racial Research* was published. Gauch argued that,

> We can advance the assertion that at the base of all Racial Science there is no concept of "human being" in contradistinction to animals separated by any physical or mental trait; the only existing differentiation is between Nordic man, on the one hand, and animals as a whole, including all non-Nordic human beings, or sub-men, who are transitional forms of development. It has not been proven, moreover, that the non-Nordic man cannot be mated with apes.[4]

However Gauch soon caused embarrassment to the leadership when he published *Out of the Flower Garden of Racial Research*, in which he went further, calling Italians "half-ape". As a result, the work was banned in Nazi Germany.[5]

He also believed that racial mixture led to disease, claiming that "Hereditary cancer is the conflict of races within the human body."[6]

Gauch also advocated de-Christianising German culture. He submitted a proposal to Darré to reform the calendar, getting rid of Christian festivals and replacing them with Germanic pagan ones. The proposal led to a protest from the future Pope Pius XII.[7] He also proposed that Charlemagne, known as Karl the Great (Karl der Grosse) in German, should be officially renamed Karl the Slaughterer, because of his wars against the pagan Saxons in the name of Christianity. He was instrumental in the creation of a memorial to pagans murdered by Charlemagne in the Massacre of Verden, which was erected in Verden an der Aller in 1935.[7]

9.3   World War II

Gauch enlisted on the outbreak of World War II, serving initially in the Luftwaffe, but was later invalided out after damaging his spine in an accident during a training flight. He subsequently claimed that he had suggested to Himmler the policy of Germanisation in Poland, by absorbing racially suitable Polish children, who showed "Nordic" characteristics.[2] On 13 October 1939 he took custody of downed RAF officer Harry Day, with whom he remained in contact after the war.[8]

He served in the Yugoslav campaign and was commended for his actions capturing Zagreb with a few men. He then became a doctor with the 23rd Luftnachrichtenregiment. Reapplying once more to the SS in 1942, his application was supported by Oswald Pohl, but he was again rejected by Himmler. He ran a hospital in Lauterecken until the final stage of the war, when he was transferred to the Western front, suffering a serious injury in the last few weeks of the conflict.[2]

9.4   Post-war

Gauch was cleared of involvement in war crimes following the denazifaction process, but could not work as a state physician. He maintained a successful private practice in Kaiserlautern.[2] According to his son, he continued to believe in his racial theories after the war, convincing himself that neo-Nazis would eventually take power in Germany. He also argued that accepted statistics of Jewish deaths in the Holocaust were highly exaggerated, and indeed impossible.[1] He was an active member of the Deutsche Reichspartei, and acted as its regional spokesman on culture and education. In 1961 he was named in the Eichmann

trial for providing ideological justification for the Holocaust because of his view that non-Nordics are "sub-human".[9]

9.5   Family

He married in 1943. His son Sigfrid was born in 1945, a few weeks before the end of the war. The couple also had a daughter. Hermann's womanising led to him separating from his wife seven years later, and he subsequently lived with a mistress.[2] Soon after his death in 1978 Sigfrid published *Vaterspuren* (1979; translated as *Traces of my Father*), a book which provided a model for later memoirs about coping with a Nazi family background.[1]

9.6   References

[1] Figge, Susan, "Father books: Memoirs of the Children of Fascist Fathers", 'Revealing Lives, Yallom and Bell, eds, pp 196-200

[2] Copley, Antony, "Hitler's Children, A Preface to Sigfid Gauch's Vaterspuren", in Gauch, Sigfrid, *Traces of My Father*, William Radice, trans. Northwestern University Press, xi-xx.

[3] Gauch, Hans (1934). *New Foundations of Racial Science*. USA: Encyclopedia of the Third Reich. p. 281. ISBN 1-56924-917-2.

[4] Stetson Kennedy, *Southern Exposure*, Doubleday, 1946, p.331

[5] "Reich Bans Book Calling Italian People Half Ape". *The New York Times*. 8 December 1934. p. 8.

[6] Hamilton Fish Armstrong, *We or They:Two Worlds in Conflict*, Macmillan, New York, 1936. p21

[7] Gauch, Sigfrid (trans. Radice, Wilhem), *Traces of my Father*, Northwestern University Press, p.92.

[8] Gauch, p.81-82.

[9] The Trial of Adolf Eichmann, Sessions 6-7-8, Nizkor Project.

Chapter 10

Hans F. K. Günther

Hans Friedrich Karl Günther (February 16, 1891 – September 25, 1968) was a German race researcher and eugenicist in the Weimar Republic and the Third Reich. He was also known as *Race Günther* (*Rassengünther*) or *Race Pope* (*Rassenpapst*). He is considered to have been a major influence on National Socialist racialist thought. He taught at the universities of Jena, Berlin, and Freiburg, writing numerous books and essays on racial theory. Günther's *Short Ethnology of the German People* (1929) was a popular exposition of Nordicism. In May 1930 he was appointed to a new chair of racial theory at Jena. He joined the Nazi Party in 1932 as the only leading racial theorist to join the party before it assumed power in 1933.[1][2]

10.1 Biography

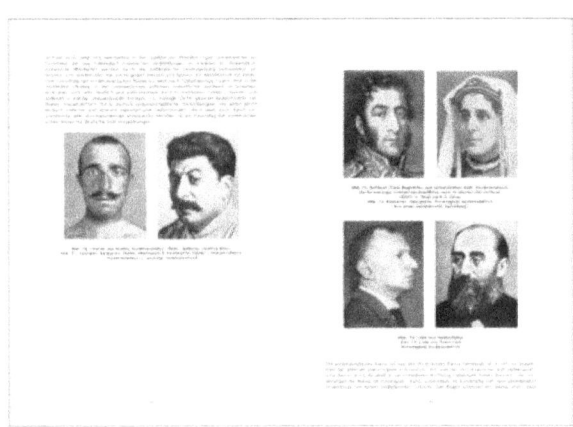

Pages 34-5 of Short Ethnology of the German People. *On the left page (right of two) there is an image of Josef Stalin as representative of the Armenoid race while on the right page (bottom two of four) there are two images of Jews from Germany and Austria respectively, described as "mainly Near Eastern", which is also known as Armenoid.*

Günther was the son of a musician. He studied comparative linguistics at Albert Ludwigs University in Freiburg, but also attended lectures on zoology and geography. In 1911,

he spent a semester at the Sorbonne, Paris. He attained his doctorate in 1914. In the same year he enlisted in the infantry at the outbreak of World War I, but became sick and was hospitalized. He was declared unfit for combat, so to compensate for his inability to fight, he served with the Red Cross.

In 1919, after the end of the war, he started his writing career. He wrote a polemical work entitled *"The Knight, death and the devil: the heroic idea"*, a reworking of the tradition of German Pagan-Nationalist Romanticism into a form of "biological nationalism". Heinrich Himmler was very impressed by this book. In 1922 Günther studied at the University of Vienna while working in a museum in Dresden. In 1923 he moved to Scandinavia to live with his second wife, who was Norwegian. He received scientific awards from the University of Uppsala and the Swedish Institute for Race Biology, headed by Herman Lundborg. In Norway he met Vidkun Quisling. In May 1930 he was appointed to the University of Jena by Wilhelm Frick who had become the first NSDAP minister in a state government when he was appointed minister of education in the right-wing coalition government formed in Thuringen following an election in December 1929. In 1935 he became a professor at the University of Berlin, teaching race science, human biology and rural ethnography. From 1940 to 1945 he was professor at Albert Ludwigs University.

He received several honors during the Third Reich, notably in 1935 he was declared "pride of the NSDAP" for his scientific work. In the same year he received the Rudolph Virchow plaque, and in 1940 the Goethe Medal for arts and science from Hitler. In March 1941, he was received as an honored guest for the opening conference of Alfred Rosenberg's "Institute for the Study of the Jewish Question". At the conference the obliteration of Jewish identity, or "people death" (*Volkstod*) of the Jews was discussed. Various proposals were made, including the "pauperization of European Jews and hard labor in massive camps in Poland". Günther's only recorded comment was that the meeting was boring.

After World War II, Günther was placed in internment

camps for three years until it was concluded that, though he was a part of the Nazi system, he was not an instigator of its criminal acts, making him less accountable for the consequences of his actions. The University of Freiburg came to his defense at his post-war trial. Nevertheless, even after Nazi Germany's fall, he did not revise his thinking, denying the Holocaust until his death. In 1951 he published the book "Husband's Choice" in which he listed good biological qualities to look for in marriage partners. He continued to argue that sterilization should remain a legal option, and played down the mandatory sterilization used in Nazi Germany. Another eugenics book was published in 1959 in which he argued that unintelligent people reproduce too numerously in Europe, and the only solution was state-sponsored family planning.

10.2 Racial theories

Günther's theories arose from the Nordicist ideology prevalent at the time. Eugen Fischer, the professor of anthropology in Freiburg, was an influential proponent of these ideas and had lectured at Albert Ludwigs University when Günther studied there.

He wrote that a race could be identified in the following manner.

> "A race shows itself in a human group which is marked off from every other human group through its own proper combination of bodily and mental characteristics, and in turn produces only its like"[3]

Günther divided the European population into six races, the Nordic, Phalic, Eastern, Western, Dinaric and East Baltic. "Western" and "Eastern" were, in practice, alternatives for the more widely used terms "Mediterranean" and "Alpine". The "Phalic" race was a minor category dropped in many of his writings.

Günther wrote in his book *Rassenkunde des deutschen Volkes* (English: *Racial Science of the German People*) he categorized the Germans as being Nordic, Mediterranean, Dinaric, Alpine and East Baltic.

Of these races, the Nordic was the noblest and was the great creative force in history. Günther claimed to have found evidence that tall, blond Nordics were the founders of influential cultures almost everywhere. Opposed to the Nordics were the Jews, who were "a thing of ferment and disturbance, a wedge driven by Asia into the European structure." Günther argued that the Nordic peoples should unite to secure their dominance.

Although Günther seemed to admire Mediterraneans and

Dinarics, as well as the highly praised Nordics, the East Baltic race was considered inferior in nearly every instance Günther mentioned it in his book, *The Racial Elements of European History*.

Among his disciples was Bruno Beger who, after an expedition to Tibet, concluded that the Tibetan peoples had characteristics that placed them between the Nordic and Mongol races, and were thus superior to other East Asians.

10.3 Influence on Hitler

Timothy Ryback, who examined the books retrieved from Adolf Hitler's private collection, notes that Hitler owned six books by Günther, four of which were different editions of *Rassenkunde des deutschen Volkes*.[4] These were given to him by Günther's publisher Julius Lehmann, who inscribed three of them. The earliest, a third edition from 1923, is for "the successful champion of German racial thinking," while the 1928 edition bears a "Christmas greeting." The 1933 sixteenth edition, with a detailed appendix on European Jews, shows signs of extended, sustained use. Lehmann dedicated it to "the trailblazer of racial thinking." Ryback notes that Hitler included Günther's book on a list of books recommended for all National Socialists to read.[5] When newly appointed Thuringian Education Minister Wilhelm Frick--the first NSDAP minister in government--appointed Günther to a chair in "Social Anthropology" at the University of Jena in 1930 (for which Jena professors considered him unqualified), Adolf Hitler and Hermann Göring demonstratively attended his inaugural lecture.[6]

10.4 See also

- Nordic theory

- Aryan race

10.5 References

[1] Alan E Steinweis. Studying the Jew: Scholarly Antisemitism in Nazi Germany. Harvard University Press, Jun 30, 2009 p.26

[2] Donna F. Ryan, John S. Schuchman. 2002. Deaf People in Hitler's Europe. Gallaudet University Press p. 19

[3] Gunther, Hans F. K., *The Racial Elements of European History*, translated by G. C. Wheeler, Methuen & Co. LTD, London, 1927, p. 3

[4] Timothy Ryback, *Hitler's Private Library: The Books that Shaped His Life* (New York: Knopf, 2008), 110.

[5] Timothy Ryback, *Hitler's Private Library: The Books that Shaped His Life* (New York: Knopf, 2008), 69. Ryback does not cite a source for this list, which may have been a book list distributed by Alfred Rosenberg's *Kampfbund für deutsche Kultur*. See Jan-Pieter Barbian, *Literaturpolitik im Dritten Reich: Institutionen, Kompetenzen, Betätigungsfelder*(Nördlingen, revised edition 1995), p. 56ff.

[6] German H.F.K Günther Wikipedia page https: //de.wikipedia.org/wiki/Hans_F._K._Günther

- Christopher Hale *Himmler's Crusade: the True Story of the 1938 Nazi Expedition into Tibet* Bantam, 2004 ISBN 978-0-553-81445-3

10.6   Further reading

- Spiro, Jonathan P. (2009). *Defending the Master Race: Conservation, Eugenics, and the Legacy of Madison Grant*. Univ. of Vermont Press. ISBN 978-1-58465-715-6. Lay summary (29 September 2010).

10.7   External links

- The Works Of HFK Günther in German and English

Chapter 11

Hans Heinze

Hans Heinze, sometimes referred to as *Euthanasie-Heinze* ("Euthanasia Heinze"; 18 October 1895 – 4 February 1983) was a Nazi German psychiatrist and eugenicist. In 1997/1998 his rehabilitation as a consequence of the request submitted by a German historian as a means of obtaining research material caused controversy.

11.1 Life

After service as a medical orderly during World War I Heinze trained as a psychiatrist at Leipzig, where he worked from 1924 in child psychiatry. He was later appointed director of the child psychiatry department of the University Clinic in Berlin, and also, in 1934, director of the *Landesheilanstalt* in Potsdam, holding the two posts simultaneously. On 2 October 1939 he was appointed Dozent for neurology and psychiatry in the medical faculty of Berlin University, where on 6 April 1943 he became a professor.

In November 1938 Heinze took over the direction of the *Landes-Pflegeanstalt Brandenburg an der Havel* mental institution, commonly now referred to as the Brandenburg Euthanasia Centre,[1] with about 2,500 patients, 1,000 of them children. Here he supervised the murder by injection, starvation and poisoning of thousands of children whose brains he then supplied to Nazi researchers.[2] He also trained physicians for the T4 Euthanasia Programme.

After the war Heinze remained in post at Brandenburg-Görden. The Russians were interested in some of his work and offered him the direction of an institution in the Crimea, but when he turned this down, tried him for war crimes, convicting him on 14 March 1946. He was imprisoned for seven years, mostly in the Soviet Special Camp No. 7 at Sachsenhausen, where he worked as the camp doctor.[3][4]

He was released on 14 March 1952 and declined offers of senior medical posts in the Volkspolizei and at the University of Jena in order to return to his family in West Germany. He took up the directorship of the department of child and adolescent psychiatry in the hospital of Wunstorf in Lower Saxony, where he remained until his retirement, and where he died in 1983.[5]

11.2 German judicial investigation

In 1962 the legal authorities of Lower Saxony opened a preliminary investigation into Heinze, but the proceedings were halted after Heinze, represented by the lawyer Kurt Giese (formerly a senior lawyer in the Private Chancellery of the Führer) was declared psychologically unfit for the process.[5]

11.3 Rehabilitation

In 1997 Dr Klaus-Dieter Müller, a German historian seeking research material, approached the Russian military authorities for their files on Heinze, which he was only able to obtain by entering a request for Heinze's rehabilitation (a recognition by the Russian authorities of Heinze's innocence of the crimes for which he had been imprisoned). As a result of Müller's request the Russian military legal service reviewed Heinze's case and in 1998 declared him rehabilitated. This caused considerable discussion in Germany of the extent to which historians should take responsibility for the consequences of their researches.[6][7]

11.4 Publications

- *Veränderungen des Liquor cerebrospinalis und ihre Bedeutung für die Auffassung vom Wesen des Ischias*, Leipzig 1923

- *Kindliche Charaktere und ihre Abartigkeiten*, Paul Schröder with explanatory case studies by Hans Heinze, Breslau 1931

- *Zur Phänomenologie des Gemüts*, Berlin 1932

- *Die Entstehung und Funktion des intervillösen Raumes*, Halle 1933

- *Rasse und Erbe: Ein Wegweiser auf dem Gebiet der Rassenkunde, Vererbungslehre und Erbgesundheitspflege für den Gebrauch an Volks- und Mittelschulen*, Halle 1934

- *'Zirkuläres Irresein (manisch-depressives): Psychopathologische Persönlichkeiten", Handbuch der Erbkrankheiten* ("Handbook of Hereditary Illnesses"), ed. Arthur Julius Gütt, Vol. 4, revised by Hans Heinze et al., Thieme, Leipzig 1942[8]

- *Ein Geschwisterpaar mit Myoklonusepilepsie*, Bonn 1955

11.5   Notes and references

[1] not the same buildings that are now Brandenburg-Görden Prison

[2] "The Rise of hatred & violence in Germany - Freedom Magazine". *Freedom Magazine*. 1995. p. 58. Retrieved April 27, 2014.

[3]

[4] p. 17, Ernst Klee: „Was sie taten – Was sie wurden", p. 136

[5] Ernst Klee: „Was sie taten – Was sie wurden", pp. 137/138

[6] „Verfolgung unterm Sowjetstern in der SBZ/DDRF", XV. Bautzen-Forum der Friedrich-Ebert-Stiftung, Büro Leipzig, 13 and 14 May 2004, ISBN 3-89892-296-0 (PDF; 695 kB)

[7] Warum ein Nazi-Massenmörder rehabilitiert wurde. *Spiegel Online, 24 August 2004]*

[8] The Deutsche Nationalbibliothek lists this 6-volume handbook of Nazi euthanasia medicine only at Leipzig, in the former DDR. In the former BRD the copies at Frankfurt/Main were apparently disposed of; in any event they are not now to be found in the OPAC.

11.6   See also

- Euthanasia

11.7   External links

- Archived version; original version link is dead: List of FBI Files on Nazi War Crimes page 2

11.8   Bibliography

- Götz Aly (ed.): *Aktion T4. 1939–1945. Die „Euthanasie"-Zentrale in der Tiergartenstraße 4.* 2nd expanded edition. Edition Hentrich, Berlin 1989, ISBN 3-926175-66-4 (*Reihe deutsche Vergangenheit. Stätten der Geschichte Berlins* 26), (exhibition catalogue)

- Henry Friedlander: *Der Weg zum NS-Genozid. Von der Euthanasie zur Endlösung.* Berlin, Berlin-Verlag 1997, ISBN 3-8270-0265-6

- Ernst Klee, ed. (1985) (in German), *Dokumente zur „Euthanasie"*, Frankfurt am Main: Fischer, ISBN 3-596-24327-0

- Ernst Klee: *„Euthanasie" im NS-Staat. Die „Vernichtung lebensunwerten Lebens".* 11th edition. Fischer-Taschenbuch-Verlag, Frankfurt am Main 2004, ISBN 3-596-24326-2 (*Fischer-Taschenbücher. 4326 Die Zeit des Nationalsozialismus*)

- Ernst Klee: *Hans Heinze.* In: Ernst Klee: *Das Personenlexikon zum Dritten Reich. Wer war was vor und nach 1945.* (updated edition). Fischer-Taschenbuch-Verlag, Frankfurt am Main 2005, ISBN 3-596-16048-0, p. 43 (*Fischer* 16048)

- Ernst Klee: *Was sie taten – was sie wurden. Ärzte, Juristen und andere Beteiligte am Kranken- oder Judenmord.* 12th edition. Fischer-Taschenbuch-Verlag, Frankfurt am Main 2004, ISBN 3-596-24364-5 (*Fischer-Taschenbücher. 4364 Die Zeit des Nationalsozialismus*)

- Ernst Klee: *Verschonte Medizinverbrecher. Die Professoren Heinze und Hallervorden.* In: *Dachauer Hefte.* 13, 1997, ISSN 0257-9472, pp. 143–152

- Alexander Mitscherlich, Fred Mielke (ed.): *Medizin ohne Menschlichkeit. Dokumente des Nürnberger Ärzteprozesse* (new edition). Fischer-Taschenbuch-Verlag, Frankfurt am Main 1987, ISBN 3-596-22003-3 (*Fischer-Taschenbücher* 2003)

- Spiegel Online, 24 August 2004@ *Warum ein Nazi-Massenmörder rehabilitiert wurde*

- Manfred Müller-Küppers: Die Geschichte der Kinder- und Jugendpsychiatrie unter besonderer Berücksichtigung der Zeit des Nationalsozialismus in: *Forum der Kinder- und Jugendpsychiatrie und Psychotherapie* Heft 2, 2001

- Hans-Walter Schmuhl: "Hirnforschung und Krankenmord. Das Kaiser-Wilhelm-Institut für Hirnforschung

1937 - 1945 (PDF; 243 kB)" Series: Ergebnisse, 1. Stand 2000

- dsb.: Medizin in der NS-Zeit: Hirnforschung und Krankenmord in: *Deutsches Ärzteblatt* 2001; Year 98. A 1240–1245, Heft 19

Chapter 12

Willibald Hentschel

Willibald Hentschel (born 7 November 1858 in Łódź - died 2 February 1947 in Berg, Upper Bavaria) was a German agrarian and volkisch writer and political activist. He sought to renew the Aryan race through a variety of schemes, including selective breeding and polygamy, all within a firmly rural setting.[1]

12.1 Early political activity

A student of biology at the University of Jena, Henstchel studied for his doctorate under celebrated Darwinist Ernst Haeckel.[2] He used his knowledge to patent an indigo dye from which he earned a fortune that enabled him to concentrate his efforts on political ventures.[2] Amongst his earliest activities was his place on the board of directors of the German Social Party, an anti-Semitic group led by Max Liebermann von Sonnenberg in the 1890s.[2] His 1901 book *Varuna*, in which he explored the supposed origins of the Aryan race, helped to make him a popular figure on the far right.[2] In this book he argued that history was driven by the process of racial purification and the energy and spirit that drove this desire.[3] Hentschel was close to Theodor Fritsch and with him founded the anti-Semitic journal *Hammer* in 1903.[1] Fritsch announced that *Varuna*, which complained that Germans were becoming "Semitized" through such initiatives as democratisation and rural depopulation, was the ideological basis of the new journal.[2]

12.2 *Mittgart*

In 1904 he published the book *Mittgart* in which he outlined a scheme to send 1000 ethnically pure women and 100 men picked for their military and athletic prowess to large country estates to procreate. Their children would then leave the estates at the age of 16 with the aim of travelling Germany and renewing racial stock.[2] He further argued that in time the countryside would be the only place were pure Germans would be found, with the cities housing the biologically unfit who would die away quickly.[4] Hentschel's scheme attracted criticism not only from religious leaders but also from fellow racial nationalists who were outraged by what they saw as an attack on the institution of the family.[2] Hentschel for his part belonged to the tendency within German nationalism that was strongly opposed to Christianity.[5] Despite the criticism he founded his own Mittgart-Bund to publicise his idea and even attempted to start his colony in Lower Saxony although this scheme met with little success and had been abandoned before 1914.[6]

12.3 Interbellum

After World War I he moderated his ideas somewhat, calling instead for a migration of ethnic Germans into the east of the country in order to displace the Poles living there.[2] Hentschel called for these Germans to be *Artamanen*, a portmanteau word he created from *art* and *manen*, Middle High German words meaning 'agriculture man' and indicating his desire for a retreat from urban life to an idyllic rural past.[7] His vision inspired the creation of the Artaman League youth movement in which the likes of Heinrich Himmler and Richard Walther Darré were active.

Hentschel joined the Nazi Party (as member number 144,649) on 1 August 1929 although, whilst his ideas about eugenics were influential on Nazism as an ideology, he had no real influence in the party personally.[8]

12.4 References

[1] Richard S. Levy, *Antisemitism: A Historical Encyclopedia of Prejudice and Persecution, Volume 1*, ABC-CLIO, 2005, p. 296

[2] Levy, *Antisemitism*, p. 297

[3] Wendy Lower, *Nazi Empire-Building and the Holocaust in Ukraine*, UNC Press Books, 2005, p. 21

[4] Daniel Gasman, *The Scientific Origins of National Socialism*, Transaction Publishers, 2004, p. 152

[5] Michael Cherlin, Halina Filipowicz, Richard L. Rudolph, *The great tradition and its legacy: the evolution of dramatic and musical theater in Austria and Central Europe*, Berghahn Books, 2004, p. 68

[6] Everett Mendelsohn, Helga Nowotny, *Nineteen Eighty-Four: Science Between Utopia and Dystopia*, Springer, 1984, p. 179

[7] Peter Padfield, *Himmler: Reichs Führer-SS*, Cassell & Co, 2001, p. 37

[8] Gregor Pelger: 'Willibald Hentschel', in Ingo Haar & Michael Fahlbusch (eds.), *Handbuch der völkischen Wissenschaften. Personen – Institutionen – Forschungsprogramme – Stiftungen*. Munich 2008, p. 243

Chapter 13

Alfred Hoche

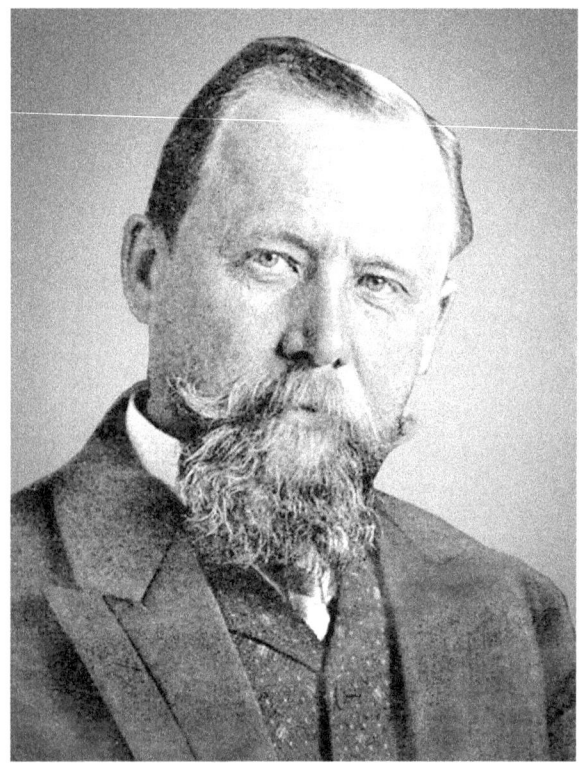

Alfred Erich Hoche sometime before 1923

Alfred Erich Hoche (German pronunciation: [ˈalfʁeːt ˈeːʁɪç ˈhɔxə]; August 1, 1865 in Wildenhain, Province of Saxony - May 16, 1943 in Baden-Baden) was a German psychiatrist well known for his writings about eugenics and euthanasia.

13.1 Life

Hoche studied in Berlin and Heidelberg and became a psychiatrist in 1890. He moved to Strasbourg in 1891. From 1902 he was a professor at Freiburg im Breisgau and was a director of the psychiatric clinic there. He was a major opponent of the psychoanalysis theories of Sigmund Freud. Hoche's body of work on the classification system of mental illness[1] had great influence.[2] He also published poetry under the pseudonym Alfred Erich.

According to Michael Burleigh's book "Death and Deliverance" he was married to a Jewish woman and left his post at Freiburg after National Socialists came to power. He was privately critical of Nazi euthanasia program after it claimed one of his relatives despite its rationale being based on his own ideas. After losing his only son in 1915 he became increasingly taciturn and depressed and his death in 1943 was probably due to suicide.[3]

13.2 Publications and Ideas

Allowing the destruction of life unworthy of living (life unworthy of life)

In Binding and Hoche's book, Hoche calls for the killing of the mentally ill and especially considers those who have been what he calls, "mentally or intellectually dead" since birth or early childhood.[4]

Hoche begins his relatively short text by reminding readers that in the society of the day (1920s Germany) deaths caused by doctors were, in some cases at least, actually taken for granted. He mentions the risk taken by patients during operations and the killing of a child during birth to save the life of a mother. Hoche stresses that none of these killings are actually legal and although a doctor can not always be sure of escaping prosecution, they are examples of where non-legal killings are accepted by the society of the day.

Hoche talks about euthanasia as proposed by Binding, arguing that if killing a person would lead to other lives being saved, it would be justifiable (Utilitarianism). Hoche believed that the killing of patients which he claimed had neither value for society, nor for themselves should be allowed.

Hoche was unable to establish an absolute rule for the first group (incurable illness) as they had not all "lost their objective and subjective value of life" and so concentrated on the second group, which he presumed had already done so. It is clear that this group would be substantially larger than the first.

Again Hoche saw an important difference in the people belonging to this group and he split it accordingly. He divided the group into people that have entered this condition later in life after "being mentally normal or at least average for a period of their life" (Dementia Paralytica/ Dementia Praecox) and in those that had either been born in the condition or where this had occurred in early childhood. Hoche argued that anyone born with this condition could never have developed any emotional relationship to their environment or family, whereas a person who had lived normally for most of their life would have had this possibility. This would enable them to display thankfulness or reverence and to connect strong memories to these feelings. This was important to take into account when deciding on a killing, yet it was not to be equated with the killing of another human being.

Hoche argued that the "mentally dead" are easily identified, they have no clear imagination, no feelings, wishes or determination. They have no possibility to develop a *Weltbild*, or a relationship to their environment. Most importantly, they lack a self-consciousness or even the possibility to become conscious of their own existence. They have no subjective claim to life, as their feelings are just simple elemental ones such as those found in the lower animals.

Hoche criticises the "modern endeavour" that has blocked "our German duty", which wants to "keep the weakest of all alive" and "has blocked attempts at preventing the mentally dead at least from procreating" and he speaks of "elements of less value", "weaklings" or "ballast existences".

Hoche then begins to argue for the killing of the disabled for purely financial reasons. Calculating the "financial and moral burden" on a person's environment, hospital and on the state, Hoche claimed that those who were "completely mentally dead" at the same time weighed heavily on "our national burden".

Binding and Hoche's book along with those by Alfred Ploetz, Rupp and Jost, directly influenced the Nazi T-4 Euthanasia Program of the 1930s. Hoche postulated "that perhaps one day we will come to the conclusion that the disposal of the mentally dead is not criminally nor morally wrong, but a useful act".

Hoche argued that the state can be seen "as an organism, as a human body which - as every doctor knows - in the interests of the survival of the whole, gives up or discards parts which have become valueless or damaging". In the case of the mentally ill these were those who were valueless and were to be discarded.

Hoche believed his ideas would be widely accepted only after, "a change in consciousness, a realisation of the unim-

portance of a single person's existence compared to that of the entirety... the absolute duty of bringing together all available energy and the feeling of belonging to a greater undertaking". Arguably this was to take place much faster than even Hoche had expected, a little more than a decade later, his ideas became part of German (Nazi) law.

13.3 Jahresringe: Innenansicht eines Menschenlebens

In his comments to the second edition of Hoche's "Jahresringe", Tilde Marchionini-Soetbeer, the book's editor, claimed that "out of love to his dead friend of 20 years", "I have taken it upon myself, with the help of understanding critics, to edit or even remove parts of the text which ... (Hoche) would have rejected, are outdated or unjust". These included Hoche's ideas "grouped around the euthanasia problem". Marchionini claimed that by 1950, Hoche would have rejected the idea, "had he experienced the inhumanities which doctors are capable of, if they are given the right to kill".

In his book, Hoche spoke about the "centuries in Germany, in which it was impossible to travel through the country, without seeing a sinner hanging from a gallows; years ago, they had stronger nerves than us and reached to the gallows more quickly. They were times in which a well trained judge was able to undertake interrogations using torture and could face the hanged and their smell as they decayed". (P195)

Hoche was interested in anatomy and took part in autopsies. He preferred people who had faced the guillotine: "because of the importance of the freshest possible material for investigation". Hoche detailed how he had taken part in at least one illegal experiment on such a person. Smuggling himself into an autopsy as an assistant to investigate the effects of electricity on the human central nervous system, Hoche connected a hidden motor to the body to see if he could make it move.

Eventually, after the state prosecution gave him special permission, Hoche was able to experiment on bodies within two minutes of their execution by guillotine. (P197)

13.4 Hoche's relevance today

Advocates of euthanasia have been accused of being influenced by Hoche, whether knowingly or not.

In particular, several authors[5][6][7][8] have drawn similarities between the arguments of Hoche and those of Australian philosopher Peter Singer.[9]

13.5   Publications

- Jahresringe.   Innenansicht eines Menschenlebens, Hoche A, 1933

- Jahresringe.   Innenansicht eines Menschenlebens, Hoche A, Lehmans Verlag, München, 1950 Hrsg. Tilde Marchionini-Soetbeer

- Die Freigabe der Vernichtung lebensunwerten Lebens. Ihr Maß und ihre Form, Binding, K. Hoche, A. 1920, 1922 Felix Meiner Verlag, Leipzig

13.6   See also

- Alfred Ploetz

- Das Recht auf den Tod, Eizabeth Rupp

- Das Recht auf den Tod, Adolf Jost

13.7   References

[1] Dening R G, Dening T R & Berrios G E (1991) Hoche and his "The Significance of Symptom Complexes in Psychiatry". *History of Psychiatry* 2: 329-343

[2] Berrios G E & Dening T R (1991) Alfred Hoche and DSM-III-R. *Biological Psychiatry* 29: 93-95

[3] Dening R G, Dening T R & Berrios G E (1991) Hoche and his "The Significance of Symptom Complexes in Psychiatry". *History of Psychiatry* 2: 329-343

[4] https://de.wikipedia.org/w/index.php?title=Datei: BindingHoche_FreigabeCoverAufl22.jpg

[5] Wright, Walter (2000). "Peter Singer and the Lessons of the German Euthanasia Program". Issues in Integrative Studies No 18, pp27-43. Available online

[6] O'Mathúna, Dónal P (March 2006). "Human dignity in the Nazi era: implications for contemporary bioethics". BMC Medical Ethics, March 2006. Available online

[7] Hendin, Herbert. "Euthanasia and Senicide". Available online

[8] Rosenblum, Jonathan (December 27, 2007). "Not a Doctor's Decision". Jerusalem Post. Available online

[9] Singer, Peter (1993). *Practical Ethics, 2nd Edition*. Cambridge. Extract available online

13.8   External links

- Works by Alfred Hoche at Project Gutenberg

- Works by or about Alfred Hoche at Internet Archive

- Life Unworthy of Life.com

Chapter 14

Max Hodann

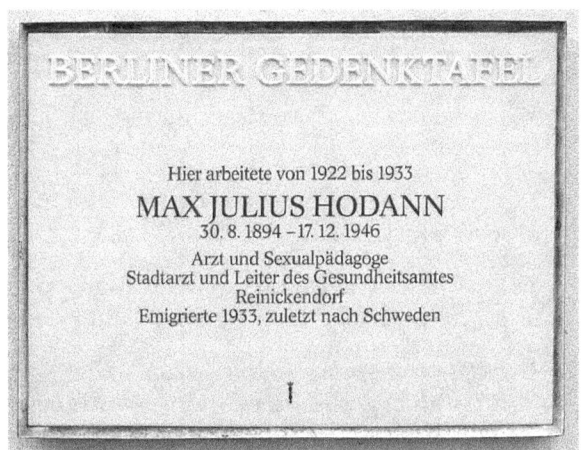

A plaque to Hodmann hanging at Reinickendorf 45, in Berlin

Max Julius Carl Alexander Hodann (30 August 1894 – 17 December 1946) was a German physician, eugenicist, sex educator and socialist, "the best-known and most controversial medical sex educationalist in the Weimar Republic".[1] He wrote for a working-class readership (e.g. *Guy and Gal*, 1924) and for children (e.g. *Where Children Come From*, 1926). After 1933, as a refugee from Nazi Germany, he lived predominantly in Norway and Sweden.

14.1 Life

Max Hodann was born in Neisse, Upper Silesia, the son of a military doctor. After his father died in 1899, Hodann and his mother moved to Berlin, then to Meran in the Tyrol, and back to Berlin in 1904. He was educated at a Berlin *gymnasium* and took part in the German Youth Movement. He studied medicine at the University of Berlin, graduating (after interruption to for army service in World War I) in 1919.[2]

Hodann was a medical health officer in Reinickendorf, Berlin from 1922 to 1923. He worked at Magnus Hirschfeld's Institute for Sexual Science from 1926 to 1929

as head of sexual counseling and the "eugenic department for mother and child" He organized public question-and-answer sex education evenings, and wrote several sex education publications which were temporarily banned. He was a member of the Association of Socialist Physicians and the National League for Birth Control and Sexual Hygiene in Weimar Germany.[3]

Hodann was arrested in February 1933, and detained without trial for several months. He crossed the border to Switzerland, staying briefly in France, the Netherlands and Denmark before living in England,[2] where he was unsuccessful in efforts to set up an Institute.[3] Moving to Norway, where he was financially supported by the Norwegian workers' organization Arbeidernes Justisfond, he published articles on family and sexuality in the Norwegian workers' press. After visiting Palestine in 1934, he co-authored a book with Lise Lindbæk about the Jewish return to Palestine. He worked as a military doctor in Spain from 1937 to 1938, returning to Norway and publishing a children's novel in Norwegian under the pseudonym **Henry M. Dawes**. Shortly before the Occupation of Norway, he moved to Sweden. There he published a novel worked with German military deserters,[2] as well as with the Swedish Association for Sex Education (RFSU).[4] He died from an asthma attack in Stockholm on 17 December 1946. There are papers at the Archives of the Swedish Municipal Workers' Union in Stockholm.[2]

14.2 Works

- (ed.) *Die Jugend zum Sexualproblem* (Young people and the sexual problem), Leipzig, 1916.

- (ed.) *Schriften zur Jugendbewegung* (Publications on the youth movement), Leipzig: Radelli & Hille, 1916.

- (ed. with Walther Koch) *Die Urburschenschaft als Jugendbewegung; in zeitgenössischen Berichten zur Jahrhundertfeier des Wartburgfestes* (The first student fraternity as a youth movement; in contemporary reports on the centenary of the Wartburg Festival), Jena: E. Diederichs, 1917

- *Die sozialhygienische Bedeutung der Beratungsstellen für Geschlechtskranke: unter besonderer Berücksichtigung der Beratungsstelle der Landesversicherungsanstalt Berlin* (The importance for social hygiene of counselling centres for venereal diseases: with special reference to the Advisory Board of the National Insurance Institute Berlin), Leipzig: Vogel, 1919.   Doctoral dissertation, Friedrich-Wilhelms-Universität Berlin

- *Deutsche Medizinische Wochenschrift*, Vol. 45, No. 50 (1919), p. 1389

- 'Aus den Parlamenten' (From parliaments), *Deutsche Medizinische Wochenschrift*, Vol. 45, No. 51 (1919), p. 1423

- 'Hygienische Maßnahmen in Sowjet-Rußland' (Hygiene measures in Soviet Russia), *Deutsche Medizinische Wochenschrift*, Vol. 45, No. 52 (1919), p. 1442-3

- *Erziehungsarbeit und Klassenkampf* (Educational work and class struggle), Jena, Thür. Verlagsanstalt und Druckerei

- *Eltern und Kleinkinder-Hygiene (Eugenik)* (Parents and toddler-hygiene (eugenics)), Leipzig: Oldenburg, 1923.

- *Bub und mädel. Gespräche unter kameraden über die geschlechterfrage* (Guy and gal. Conversations among comrades on the gender question), Leipzig: Oldenburg, 1924. Foreword by Paul Oestreich.

  - Translated by Boris Osipovich Finkel′shteĭn into Russian, 1925; translated into Ukrainian, 1925.

  - Translated into Swedish as *Saker som man inte talar om* (Things we don't talk about), Stockholm: Arbetarkultur, 1934.

- (ed. with Heinrich Müller) *Der jugendliche Mensch und der Erzieher* (The young man and the educator), Berlin, 1925.

- *Woher die Kinden kommen: Ein Lehrbuch, für Kinder lesbar* (Where babies come from: a texbook for children to read), Rudolstadt: Greifenverlag, 1926. Illustrated by Willi Geißler. New edition (1928) as *Bringt uns wirklich der Klapperstorch? : Ein Lehrbuch, für Kinder lesbar* (Does the stork really bring us? A textbook for children to read)

- *Geschlecht und Liebe in biologischer und gesellschaftlicher Beziehung* (Sex and love in their biological and social relationship), Rudolstadt: Greifenverl., 1927.

- Translated by Jerome Gibbs as *Sex life in Europe: a biological and sociological survey*, New York: The Gargoyle Press, 1932.

- *Der Mensch, sein Körper und seine Lebenstätigkeit* (Man: his body and his life activity), München: Birk, 1927.

- *Sexualpädagogik: Erziehungshygiene und Gesundheitspolitik. Gesammelte Aufsätze u. Vortr. (1916–1927)* (Sex education: hygiene education and health policies), Rudolstadt/Thür.: Greifenverl., 1928.

- *Elternhygiene : Eugenik für Erzieher* (Parental hygiene: eugenics for educators), Rudolstadt: Greifenverl., 1928.

- *Von der Kunst des Liebesverkehrs*, Rudolstadt i. Thür.: Greifenverl., 1928

- *Die Sexualnot der Erwachsenen* (The sexual frustration of adults), Rudolstadt: Greifenverl., 1928.

- *Sexualelend und Sexualberatung* (Sexual misery and sexual counselling), Thür. Rudolstadt, 1928

- *Unzucht! Unzucht! Herr Staatsanwalt! zur Naturgeschichte des deutschen Schamgefühls* (Fornication! Fornication! Mr. Prosecutor! The natural history of German shame), Rudolstadt: Greifenverlag, 1928

- *Onanie: weder laster noch krankheit* (Masturbation: neither wicked nor illness), Berlin: Universitas, 1929

- *Sowjetunion : Gestern, Heute, Morgen* (Soviet Union: yesterday, today, tomorrow), Berlin: Universitas, 1931

- *Der slawische Gürtel um Deutschland; Polen, die Tschechoslowakei und die deutschen Ostprobleme* (The Slavic girdle of Germany: Poland, Czechoslovakia and the problem of the German East), Berlin: Universitas, 1932

- (with Lise Lindbaek) *Jødene vender hjem* (Jews returning home), Oslo: Aschehoug, 1934.

- (ed.) *The New Birth Control and Abortion Law in Iceland. (10 December 1934.) Reprinted from the Marriage Hygiene, etc.*, Bombay, 1936.

- *Sex and Modern Morality. Reprinted from the "Marriage Hygiene," etc.*, Bombay, 1936. Translated by Stella Browne.

- *History of modern morals*, London, W. Heinemann ltd, 1937. Translated by Stella Browne from the unpublished German original.

- (as Henry M. Dawes) *Jakob går over grensen*, Oslo: Tiden Norsk Forlag, 1938.

14.3 References

[1] Lutz D. H. Sauerteig (1999). "Sex education in Germany from the eighteenth to the twentieth century". In Franx X. Eder, Lesley Hall & Gert Hekma. *Sexual Cultures in Europe: Themes in Sexuality*. Manchester University Press. pp. 21–2. ISBN 978-0-7190-5321-4. Retrieved 18 December 2012.

[2] Zlata Fuss Phillips (2001). *German Children's and Youth Literature in Exile 1933–1950: Biographies and Bibliographies*. Walter de Gruyter. pp. 55–6. ISBN 978-3-11-095285-8. Retrieved 18 December 2012.

[3] Online-Exhibition by the Magnus-Hirschfield Society

[4] Lena Lenerhed (2009). "Taking the Middle Way: Sex Education Debates in Sweden in the Early Twentieth Century". In Lutz D. H. Sauerteig & Roger Davidson. *Shaping sexual knowledge: a cultural history of sex education in 20th century Europe*. Taylor & Francis. pp. 60–1. ISBN 978-0-415-41114-1. Retrieved 18 December 2012.

14.4 Further reading

- Wilfried Heinzelmann, *Sozialhygiene als Gesundheitswissenschaft : die deutsch/deutsch-jüdische Avantgarde 1897–1933 : eine Geschichte in sieben Profilen*, Bielefeld: Transcript, 2009.

- Wilfried Wolff, *Max Hodann (1894–1946): Sozialist und Sexualreformer*, 1994

Chapter 15

Fritz Lenz

Fritz A Lenz (9 March 1887 in Pflugrade, Pomerania – 6 July 1976 in Göttingen, Lower Saxony) was a German geneticist, member of the Nazi Party,[1] and influential specialist in eugenics during the Third Reich.

15.1 Biography

The pupil of Alfred Ploetz, Lenz took over the publication of the magazine "Archives for Racial and Social Biology" from 1913 to 1933 and received in 1923 the first chair in eugenics in Munich. In 1933 he came to Berlin where he established the first specific department devoted to eugenics, at the Kaiser Wilhelm Institute of Anthropology, Human Heredity, and Eugenics.

Lenz specialised in the field of the transmission of hereditary human diseases and "racial health". The results of his research were published in 1921 and 1932 in collaboration with Erwin Baur and Eugen Fischer in two volumes that were later combined under the title *Human Heredity Theory and Racial Hygiene* (1936).

This work and his theory of "race as a value principle" placed Lenz and his two colleagues in the position of Germany's leading racial theorists. Their ideas provided scientific justification for Nazi ideology, in particular its emphasis on the superiority of the "Nordic race" and the desirability of eliminating allegedly inferior strains of humanity - or "life unworthy of life" (*Lebensunwertes Leben*). Lenz was a member of the "Committee of Experts for Population and Racial Policy". He joined the Nazi party in 1937 while serving as the head of the Kaiser Wilhelm Institute for Anthropology.[1]

After World War II, Lenz continued to work as a Professor of genetics at the University of Goettingen. When questioned Lenz said that the Holocaust would undermine the study of human genetics and racial theory. He continued to believe that eugenic theories of racial differences had been scientifically proven.

15.2 Theories

For Lenz, human genetics established that the connection between racial identity and human nature was actually physical in character. This extended to political affiliations. Lenz even claimed that the revolutionary agitation in Germany after 1918 was caused by inferior racial elements, warning that the nation's racial superiority was threatened. He stated that "The German nation is the last refuge of the Nordic race...before us lies the greatest task of world history".[2] For Lenz, this validated the racialised politics of the Nazis.

He justified the Nuremberg laws of 1935 in this way:

> As important as the external features for their evaluation is the lineage of individuals, a blond Jew is also a Jew. Yes, there are Jews who have most of the external features of the Nordic race, but who nevertheless display Jewish mental tendencies. The legislation of the National Socialist state therefore properly defines a Jew not by external race characteristics, but by descent.[3]

Likewise, Lenz took the view that Slavs were inferior to Nordic peoples, and that they threatened to "overrun the superior Volk (People)." In 1940, Lenz advised the SS that "The resettlement of the Eastern zone is...the most consequential task of racial policy. It will determine the racial character of the population living there for centuries to come."

15.3 References

[1] "Human biodiversity: genes, race, and history", Jonathan M. Marks. Transaction Publishers, 1995. p. 88. ISBN 0-202-02033-9, ISBN 978-0-202-02033-4.

[2] Geoffrey G. Field, "Nordic Racism", *Journal of the History of Ideas*, University of Pennsylvania Press, 1977, p. 526

[3] Fritz Lenz, *Über Wege und Irrwege rassenkundlicher Untersuchungen*, in: *Zeitschrift für Morphologie und Anthropologie* Bd. 39, 3/1941, S. 397

15.4 See also

- Racial policy of Nazi Germany

- Eugenics

- Ex-Nazis

- Alfred Ploetz

- Ernst Rudin

- Eugen_Fischer

- racial hygiene

- Kaiser Wilhelm Institute of Anthropology, Human Heredity, and Eugenics

Chapter 16

Karin Magnussen

Karin Magnussen (9 February 1908 – 19 February 1997) was a German biologist, teacher and researcher at the Kaiser Wilhelm Institute of Anthropology, Human Heredity, and Eugenics during the Third Reich. She is known for her 1936 publication "Race and Population Policy Tools", and her studies of heterochromia iridis (different-colored eyes) using iris specimens, supplied by Josef Mengele, from Auschwitz concentration camp victims.[1]

16.1 Early life and education

Karin Magnussen, daughter of the landscape painter and ceramist Walter Magnussen, grew up with her sister in a middle-class home. She completed her schooling in Bremen, graduating with a degree. She then studied biology, geology, chemistry and physics at the University of Göttingen. Magnussen joined the National Socialist German Students' League (NSDStB) while she was still an undergraduate in college. By 1931, when she was 23, she was a member of the National Socialist German Workers Party. Later she became a leader of the League of German Girls (Bund Deutscher Mädel, or BDM) and a member of the National Socialist Teachers League. As a BDM leader, she held lectures on the politics of race and population. She graduated in 1932 with an examination in the subjects of botany, zoology and geology. In July 1932, her thesis was accepted: *Studies on the physiology of the butterfly wing*.[1]

After receiving her doctorate, she studied at the Zoological Institute of the University of Göttingen in Alfred Kühn. She placed first and later second on her state exam for a high school teaching position; *inter alia* in biology in 1936. In Hanover, Magnussen was employed as a teacher at a secondary school. Magnussen possibly modeled herself after "...the biologist Agnes Bluhm, who worked at the Kaiser-Wilhelm-Institut fur Biologie and wrote "Die rassenhygienischen Aufgaben des weiblichen Arztes", Berlin, 1934, and who unhesitatingly supported Hitler's regime." In 1935, Magnussen went to work in the Nazi Racial Policy Office in the District of Hanover. A year later, she wrote *Race and Population Policy Tools*.[1]

16.2 National Socialist views

Magnussen had already joined the National Socialist German Student League (NSDStB) during her studies. In 1931, she became a member of the NSDAP. Later, she became BDM leader and was a member of the National Socialist Teachers League (NSLB).[2] In Bremen, she lectured on racism and demographics. Magnussen was BDM leader in the Gau. In 1935, she was employed in the Gau Hannover in the Racial Politics Office.[3] Her publication of racial and folkisch political tools appeared in 1936.[2] In 1939, this script was used by Lehmann of Munich. After the end of the Second World War, in the Soviet zone of occupation, it appeared on the list of prohibited literature.[4]

In the third published edition of 1943, Magnussen expressed the following:

> "This war is not just about the preservation of the German people, but is about the question, which races and peoples should live in the future on European soil.... Basically England had no interest in the prosecution of this war, but it is a very different people, working parasitically behind the scenes and which is afraid to lose everything. In all of the enemy States, Judaism has significant influence. And just as Judaism had probably the clearest recognition that in the decisive struggle, the question of them was to be decided. The current war must therefore be also about the repression of the black danger in the West and the elimination of the Bolshevik threat in the East, which still resolves a racial problem in Europe, which all States are more or less interested in: the Jewish question. Also the Jew who enjoys life as a host in our country, is our enemy, even if he does not actively engage with weapons in this fight. ...From the European point of view,

the Jewish question is resolved in that the emigre Jews do the thinking for the leaders in the other States. We have seen that these emigrants are only troublesome and set up the peoples against each other."[5]

16.3 Kaiser Wilhelm Institute

Due to receiving a scholarship, Magnussen was suspended in the fall of 1941 from her teaching profession and moved to the Kaiser Wilhelm Institute of Anthropology, Human Heredity, and Eugenics (KWI-A), in Berlin-Dahlem.[6] From this time on, she worked in the Department of Experimental Pathology of Heritage under the Department head, Hans Nachtsheim. Her research focused on the inheritance of eye color in rabbits and humans.[7] Her particular interest was the Heterochromic iris that she had examined since 1938. Magnussen used the scientific method to lead her to the conclusion that the eye is not only genetically, but also hormonally-determined. While there, she initially undertook studies on rabbit eyes.[8] In July 1943, she was the research assistant of Otmar Freiherr von Verschuer, at the KWI-A.[6] At the KWI-A she also met Dr Mengele, who worked there temporarily.

The Deutsche Forschungsgemeinschaft (DFG) promoted her study to "explore the heritage conditionality for the development of eye color as a basis for racial and ethnicity studies" in 1943, in addition to eight other research projects at the KWI-A. This project was overseen and the publication edited by Magnussen.[9][10]

16.4 Auschwitz-Birkenau

From a colleague, she received the information that more twins and family members with Heterochromic irises would be found in the Sinti family in Mechau from northern Germany. Members of the family were taken in the spring of 1943 to the KWI-A, where they were photographed. In March 1943, the Sinti family in the Auschwitz concentration camp was deported, where Mengele had worked since late May 1943 as camp physician. This circumstance allowed Mengele to carry out the experiments (that Magnussen had done on rabbits) on the people.

According to a statement by Magnussen, Mengele dealt, among other things, with the eyes of these Sinti family using hormonal substances. Often, these painful interventions resulted in suppuration of the eyes and blindness of the victims. These experiments aimed at the investigation and eradication of the abnormality in people with Heterochromic Irises. In the event of death of the prison-

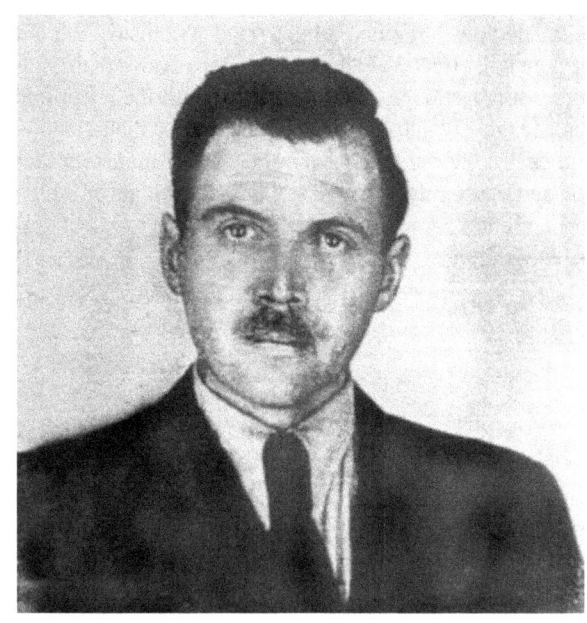

Josef Mengele in 1956. Photo taken by a police photographer in Buenos Aires for Mengele's Argentine identification document.

ers, Mengele pledged to Magnussen to give her the eyes of the victims for further research and evaluation.[11] In the second half of 1944, Magnussen received the eyes of the experiment victims from Auschwitz-Birkenau in several deliveries.[12] No fewer than 40 pairs of eyes should have been received by Magnussen from Auschwitz-Birkenau.[13] The Hungarian prisoner pathologist Miklós Nyiszli noted after the autopsy of Sinti twins that they had been killed, not due to illness, but because of a chloroform injection to the heart. Nyiszli had to prepare their eyes and send them to the KWI-A.[11]

16.5 After the war

At least until the spring of 1945, Magnussen was working in Berlin.[14] After the end of the Second World War, Magnussen moved to Bremen again and continued her research. Her completed research was published in 1949, being entitled *"On the relationship between histological distribution of pigment, Iris color and pigmentation of the eyeball of the human eye."*[15] She was later denazified in Bremen.

In 1950, Magnussen taught at a girls' high school in Bremen. She worked as study counselor and official, including the teaching of biology. She was considered a popular teacher who led an interesting biology lesson. Magnussen's pupils could examine, for example, living and dead rabbits from their breeding. Until 1964, essays in scientific journals were published by Magnussen. Magnussen retired in August 1970. Even in old age, Magnussen justified the Nazi racial ideology. She noted in 1980, in a conversation with the geneticist Benno Müller-Hill, that the Nuremberg Laws were not fair enough. She also denied until the last minute that Mengele would have killed children for their scientific studies.[16] She was entangled by her cooperation with Mengele and the supply of "human material", and mired deep in concentration camp crimes, but she claimed to know nothing about them.

In 1990, Magnussen moved into a nursing home; she died in February 1997 in Bremen.

16.6   Further reading

- Wolfgang Schieder, Achim Trunk: *Adolf Butenandt and the Kaiser-Wilhelm-Gesellschaft*. Science, industry and politics in the Third Reich. Series: History of the Kaiser-Wilhelm Gesellschaft IM Nationalsozialismus, 7 Hg. Max Planck Society for the advancement of science, Wallenstein, Göttingen 2004, ISBN 978-3-89244-423-7

- Hans Hesse: *Eyes from Auschwitz. A lesson in National Socialist racial delusion and medical research. The case of Dr. Karin Magnussen*, plain text, Essen 2001, ISBN 3-89861-009-8

- Sascha Hönighaus: "Karin Magnussen", in: Jessica Hoffman, Anja Megel, Robert Parzer & Helena Seidel eds.: *Dahlemer Memorial locations*, Frank & Timme Verlag for scientific literature, Berlin 2007, ISBN 978-3-86596-144-0

- Ernst Klee: *the person lexicon to the Third Reich: who was what before and after 1945?* Fischer, Frankfurt 2007, ISBN 3-596-16048-0 DSB.: Auschwitz, NAZI medicine and its victims. 3rd Edition. S. Fischer, Frankfurt 1997, ISBN 3-596-14906-1

- Carola Sachse Ed.: *the link to Auschwitz. Life sciences and human experiments at Kaiser-Wilhelm-Instituts*. Documentation of a symposium. Wallenstein, Göttingen 2003 series: history of the Kaiser-Wilhelm-Gesellschaft IM Nationalsozialismus, 6. ISBN 3-89244-699-7 (interim report see Web links)

- Hans-Walter Schmuhl: Grenzüberschreitungen. *Das Kaiser-Wilhelm-Institut für Anthropologie, menschliche Erblehre und Eugenik 1927–1945. Reihe: Geschichte der Kaiser-Wilhelm-Gesellschaft im Nationalsozialismus*, 9. Wallstein, Göttingen 2005, ISBN 3-89244-799-3

16.7   References

[1] "Eugenics - Karin Magnussen". Esther M. Zimmer Lederberg Memorial Website.

[2] Ernst Klee: *Das Personenlexikon zum Dritten Reich*, Frankfurt am Main 2007, p. 387

[3] Sascha Hönighaus: *Karin Magnussen*, Berlin 2007, p. 193f.

[4] Deutsche Verwaltung für Volksbildung in der sowjetischen Besatzungszone, *Liste der auszusondernden Literatur*, Berlin: Zentralverlag, 1946

[5] From her book *Rassen- und bevölkerungspolitisches Rüstzeug*. 3. Aufl. Lehmanns, München 1943, p. 201-203. *Mit "Schwarze Gefahr" sind vermutlich Afrikaner gemeint, vgl. Rheinlandbastarde, ein beliebtes NS-Feindbild*

[6] Ernst Klee: *Das Personenlexikon zum Dritten Reich*, Frankfurt am Main 2007, p. 387.

[7] Wolfgang Schieder, Achim Trunk: *Adolf Butenandt und die Kaiser-Wilhelm-Gesellschaft: Wissenschaft, Industrie und Politik im Dritten Reich*, Göttingen 2004, p. 297f.

[8] Sascha Hönighaus: *Karin Magnussen*, Berlin 2007, p. 195

[9] Hans Hesse: "Ich konnte nicht auf die Auswertung eines so wertvollen Materials verzichten - Augen aus Auschwitz: Das Kaiser-Wilhelm-Institut für Anthropologie und der Fall Karin Magnussen", *WeltOnline*, 31 August 2001

[10] Hans-Walter Schmuhl: *Grenzüberschreitungen. Das Kaiser-Wilhelm-Institut für Anthropologie, menschliche Erblehre und Eugenik 1927–1945. Geschichte der Kaiser-Wilhelm-Gesellschaft im Nationalsozialismus*, Vol. 9. Wallstein, Göttingen 2005, p. 370

[11] Rolf Winau: *Medizinische Exeperimente in Konzentrationslagern*, Wolfgang Benz, Barbara Distel (Hrsg.): *Der Ort des Terrors – Geschichte der nationalsozialistischen Konzentrationslager*, Vol. 1: Die Organisation des Terrors, C.H. Beck, München 2005, ISBN 3-406-52961-5, p. 174.

[12] Ilkka Remes: *Das Erbe des Bösen*, p. 3 (pdf).

[13] Sascha Hönighaus: *Karin Magnussen*, Berlin 2007, p. 197

[14] Ernst Klee: *Auschwitz, die NS-Medizin und ihre Opfer*, Frankfurt am Main 1997, p. 486.

[15] Hans-Walter Schmuhl: *Grenzüberschreitungen. Das Kaiser-Wilhelm-Institut für Anthropologie, menschliche Erblehre und Eugenik 1927–1945. Geschichte der Kaiser-Wilhelm-Gesellschaft im Nationalsozialismus*, Vol. 9 Wallstein, Göttingen 2005, p. 490

[16] Sascha Hönighaus: *Karin Magnussen*, Berlin 2007, p. 199f.

16.8 External links

- Literature by and about Karin Magnussen in the German National Library catalogue

- Online Magnussen passim. Verf. Carola Sachse & Benoit Massin. Stand: 2000 (Vorläuf. Ergebnisse)

- Estherlederberg

Chapter 17

Josef Mengele

"Mengele" redirects here. For other uses, see Mengele (disambiguation).

Josef Mengele (German: [ˈjoːzɛf ˈmɛŋələ]; 16 March 1911 – 7 February 1979) was a German *Schutzstaffel* (SS) officer and physician in Auschwitz concentration camp during World War II. Mengele was a notorious member of the team of doctors responsible for the selection of victims to be killed in the gas chambers and for performing deadly human experiments on prisoners. Arrivals deemed able to work were admitted into the camp, and those deemed unfit for labor were immediately killed in the gas chambers. Mengele left Auschwitz on 17 January 1945, shortly before the arrival of the liberating Red Army troops. After the war, he fled to South America, where he evaded capture for the rest of his life.

Mengele received doctorates in anthropology and medicine from Munich University and began a career as a researcher. He joined the Nazi Party in 1937 and the SS in 1938. Initially assigned as a battalion medical officer at the start of World War II, he transferred to the concentration camp service in early 1943 and was assigned to Auschwitz. There he saw the opportunity to conduct genetic research on human subjects. His subsequent experiments, focusing primarily on twins, had no regard for the health or safety of the victims.[2][3]

Assisted by a network of former SS members, Mengele sailed to Argentina in July 1949. He initially lived in and around Buenos Aires, then fled to Paraguay in 1959 and Brazil in 1960 while being sought by West Germany, Israel, and Nazi hunters such as Simon Wiesenthal so that he could be brought to trial. In spite of extradition requests by the West German government and clandestine operations by Mossad (the Israeli intelligence agency), Mengele eluded capture. He drowned while swimming off the Brazilian coast in 1979 and was buried under a false name. His remains were disinterred and positively identified by forensic examination in 1985.

17.1 Early life and education

Mengele was born the eldest of three children on 16 March 1911 to Karl and Walburga (Hupfauer) Mengele in Günzburg, Bavaria, Germany.[4] His younger brothers were Karl Jr and Alois. Mengele's father was founder of the Karl Mengele & Sons company, producers of farm machinery.[5] Mengele did well in school and developed an interest in music, art, and skiing.[6] He completed high school in April 1930 and went on to study medicine at Goethe University Frankfurt and philosophy at the University of Munich.[7] Munich was the headquarters of the Nazi Party.[8] In 1931 Mengele joined the *Stahlhelm, Bund der Frontsoldaten*, a paramilitary organisation that was in 1934 absorbed into the Nazi *Sturmabteilung* (Storm Detachment; SA).[9][7]

In 1935, Mengele earned a PhD in anthropology from the University of Munich.[7] In January 1937, at the Institute for Hereditary Biology and Racial Hygiene in Frankfurt, he became the assistant to Dr. Otmar Freiherr von Verschuer, a scientist conducting genetics research, with a particular interest in twins.[7] As an assistant to von Verschuer, Mengele focused on the genetic factors resulting in a cleft lip and palate or cleft chin.[10] His thesis on the subject earned him a *cum laude* doctorate in medicine in 1938.[11] Both of his degrees were later rescinded by the issuing universities.[12] In a letter of recommendation, von Verschuer praised Mengele's reliability and his ability to verbally present complex material in a clear manner.[13] The American author Robert Jay Lifton notes that Mengele's published works did not deviate much from the scientific mainstream of the time, and would probably have been viewed as valid scientific efforts even outside the borders of Nazi Germany.[13]

On 28 July 1939, Mengele married Irene Schönbein, whom he had met while working as a medical resident in Leipzig.[14] Their only son, Rolf, was born in 1944.[15]

17.2 Military service

The ideology of Nazism brought together elements of antisemitism, racial hygiene, and eugenics, and combined them with pan-Germanism and territorial expansionism with the goal of obtaining more *Lebensraum* (living space) for the Germanic people.[16] Nazi Germany attempted to obtain this new territory by attacking Poland and the Soviet Union, intending to deport or kill the Jews and Slavs living there, who were viewed as being inferior to the Aryan master race.[17]

Mengele joined the Nazi Party in 1937 and the *Schutzstaffel* (SS; protection squadron) in 1938. He received basic training in 1938 with the *Gebirgsjäger* (mountain infantry) and was called up for service in the Wehrmacht (German armed forces) in June 1940, some months after the outbreak of World War II. He soon volunteered for medical service in the *Waffen-SS*, the combat arm of the SS, where he served with the rank of SS-*Untersturmführer* (second lieutenant) in a medical reserve battalion until November 1940. He was next assigned to the *SS-Rasse- und Siedlungshauptamt* (SS Race and Resettlement Main Office) in Posen, evaluating candidates for Germanisation.[18][19]

In June 1941, Mengele was posted to Ukraine, where he was awarded the Iron Cross Second Class. In January 1942 he joined the 5th SS Panzer Division Wiking as a battalion medical officer. He rescued two German soldiers from a burning tank and was awarded the Iron Cross First Class, as well as the Wound Badge in Black and the Medal for the Care of the German People. He was seriously wounded in action near Rostov-on-Don in mid-1942 and was declared unfit for further active service. After recovery, he was transferred to the Race and Resettlement Office in Berlin. He also resumed his association with von Verschuer, who was at the Kaiser Wilhelm Institute for Anthropology, Human Genetics and Eugenics. Mengele was promoted to the rank of SS-*Hauptsturmführer* (captain) in April 1943.[20][21][22]

17.3 Auschwitz

In early 1943, encouraged by von Verschuer, Mengele applied for transfer to the concentration camp service, where he foresaw the opportunity to undertake genetic research on human subjects.[20][23] His application was accepted, and he was posted to Auschwitz concentration camp. He was appointed by SS-*Standortarzt* Eduard Wirths, chief medical officer at Auschwitz, to the position of chief physician of the *Zigeunerfamilienlager* (Romani family camp), located in the sub-camp at Birkenau.[20][23]

By late 1941 Hitler decided that the Jews of Europe were

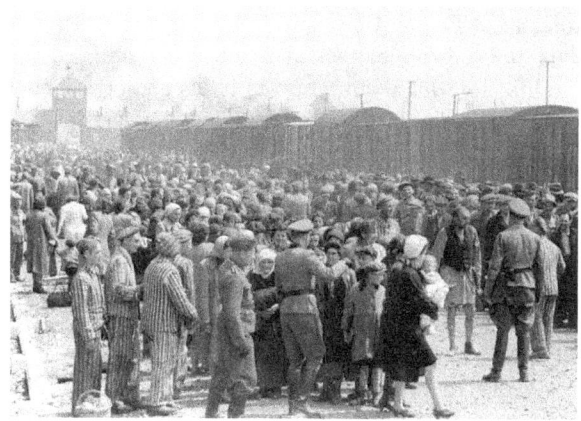

"Selection" of Hungarian Jews on the ramp at Auschwitz-II (Birkenau), May/June 1944

to be exterminated, so Birkenau, originally intended to house slave laborers, was re-purposed as a combination labor camp / extermination camp.[24][25] Prisoners were transported there by rail from all over German-occupied Europe, arriving in daily convoys.[26] By July 1942, the SS were conducting "selections". Incoming Jews were segregated; those deemed able to work were admitted into the camp, and those deemed unfit for labor were immediately killed in the gas chambers.[27] The group selected to die, about three-quarters of the total,[lower-alpha 1] included almost all children, women with small children, pregnant women, all the elderly, and all those who appeared on brief and superficial inspection by an SS doctor not to be completely fit.[29][30] Mengele, a member of the team of doctors assigned to do selections, undertook this work even when he was not assigned to do so in the hope of finding subjects for his experiments.[31] He was particularly interested in locating sets of twins.[32] In contrast to most of the doctors, who viewed undertaking selections as one of their most stressful and horrible duties, Mengele undertook the task with a flamboyant air, often smiling or whistling a tune.[33][34]

Mengele and other SS doctors did not treat inmates, but supervised the activities of inmate doctors forced to work in the camp medical service.[34] Mengele made weekly visits to the hospital barracks and sent to the gas chambers any prisoners who had not recovered after two weeks in bed.[35] He was also a member of the team of doctors responsible for supervising the administration of Zyklon B, the cyanide-based pesticide that was used to kill people in the gas chambers at Birkenau. He served in this capacity at the gas chambers located in crematoria IV and V.[36]

When an outbreak of noma (a gangrenous bacterial disease of the mouth and face) broke out in the Romani camp in 1943, Mengele initiated a study to determine the cause of the disease and develop a treatment. He enlisted the aid of prisoner Dr. Berthold Epstein, a Jewish pediatrician and professor at Prague University. Mengele isolated the patients in a separate barrack and had several afflicted children killed so that their preserved heads and organs could be sent to the SS Medical Academy in Graz and other facilities for study. The research was still ongoing when the Romani camp was liquidated and its remaining occupants killed in 1944.[2]

In response to a typhus epidemic in the women's camp, Mengele cleared one block of 600 Jewish women and sent them to the gas chamber. The building was then cleaned and disinfected, and the occupants of a neighboring block were bathed, de-loused, and given new clothing before being moved into the clean block. The process was repeated until all the barracks were disinfected. Similar disinfections were used for later epidemics of scarlet fever and other diseases, but with all the sick prisoners being sent to the gas chambers. For his efforts, Mengele was awarded the War Merit Cross (Second Class with Swords) and was promoted in 1944 to First Physician of the Birkenau subcamp.[37]

17.3.1 Human experimentation

Mengele used Auschwitz as an opportunity to continue his anthropological studies and research on heredity, using inmates for human experimentation.[2] The experiments had no regard for the health or safety of the victims.[2][3] He was particularly interested in identical twins, people with heterochromia iridum (eyes of two different colours), dwarfs, and people with physical abnormalities.[2] A grant was provided by the *Deutsche Forschungsgemeinschaft*, applied for by von Verschuer, who received regular reports and shipments of specimens from Mengele. The grant was used to build a pathology laboratory attached to Crematorium II at Auschwitz II-Birkenau.[38] Dr. Miklós Nyiszli, a Hungarian Jewish pathologist who arrived in Auschwitz on 29 May 1944, performed dissections and prepared specimens for shipment in this laboratory.[39] Mengele's twin research was in part intended to prove the supremacy of heredity over environment and thus bolster the Nazi premise of the superiority of the Aryan race.[40] Nyiszli and others report that the twins studies may also have been motivated by a desire to improve the reproduction rate of the German race by improving the chances of racially desirable people having twins.[41]

Mengele's research subjects were better fed and housed than other prisoners and temporarily safe from the gas chambers.[42] He established a kindergarten for children that were the subjects of experiments, along with all Romani children under the age of six. The facility provided better food and living conditions than other areas of the camp, and even included a playground.[43] When visiting his child subjects, he introduced himself as "Uncle Mengele"

and offered them sweets.[44] But he was also personally responsible for the deaths of an unknown number of victims that he killed via lethal injection, shootings, beatings, and through selections and deadly experiments.[45] Lifton describes Mengele as sadistic, lacking empathy, and extremely antisemitic, believing the Jews should be eliminated entirely as an inferior and dangerous race.[46] Mengele's son Rolf said his father later showed no remorse for his wartime activities.[47]

A former Auschwitz prisoner doctor said:

> He was capable of being so kind to the children, to have them become fond of him, to bring them sugar, to think of small details in their daily lives, and to do things we would genuinely admire ... And then, next to that, ... the crematoria smoke, and these children, tomorrow or in a half-hour, he is going to send them there. Well, that is where the anomaly lay.[48]

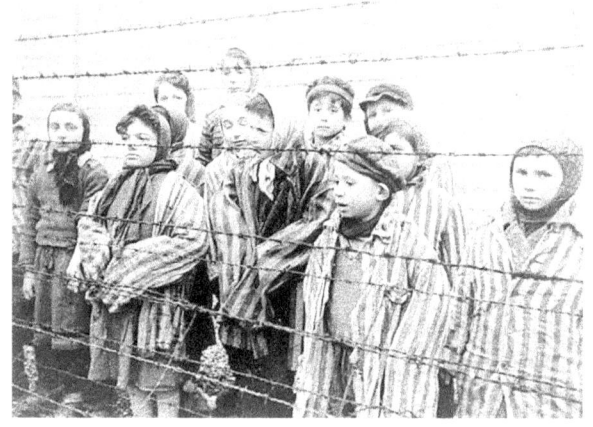

Jewish twins kept alive to be used in Mengele's medical experiments. These children were liberated from Auschwitz by the Red Army in January 1945.

Twins were subjected to weekly examinations and measurements of their physical attributes by Mengele or one of his assistants.[49] Experiments performed by Mengele on twins included unnecessary amputation of limbs, intentionally infecting one twin with typhus or other diseases, and transfusing the blood of one twin into the other. Many of the victims died while undergoing these procedures.[50] After an experiment was over, the twins were sometimes killed and their bodies dissected.[51] Nyiszli recalled one occasion where Mengele personally killed fourteen twins in one night via a chloroform injection to the heart.[34] If one twin died of disease, Mengele killed the other so that comparative post-mortem reports could be prepared.[52]

Mengele's experiments with eyes included attempts to change eye color by injecting chemicals into the eyes of living subjects and killing people with heterochromatic eyes so that the eyes could be removed and sent to Berlin for study.[53] His experiments on dwarfs and people with physical abnormalities included taking physical measurements, drawing blood, extracting healthy teeth, and treatment with unnecessary drugs and X-rays.[3] Many of the victims were sent to the gas chambers after about two weeks, and their skeletons were sent to Berlin for further study.[54] Mengele sought out pregnant women, on whom he would perform experiments before sending them to the gas chambers.[55] Witness Vera Alexander described how he sewed two Romani twins together back to back in an attempt to create conjoined twins.[50] The children died of gangrene after several days of suffering.[56]

17.4   After Auschwitz

Along with several other Auschwitz doctors, Mengele transferred to Gross-Rosen concentration camp in Lower Silesia on 17 January 1945. He brought along two boxes of specimens and records of his experiments. Most of the camp medical records had already been destroyed by the SS.[57][58] The Red Army captured Auschwitz on 27 January.[59] Mengele fled Gross Rosen on 18 February, a week before the Soviets arrived, and traveled westward disguised as a Wehrmacht officer to Saaz (now Žatec). Here he temporarily entrusted his incriminating Auschwitz documents to a nurse with whom he had struck up a relationship.[57] He and his unit hurried west to avoid being captured by the Soviets and were taken prisoner of war by the Americans in June. Mengele was initially registered under his own name, but because of the disorganization of the Allies regarding the distribution of wanted lists and the fact that Mengele did not have the usual SS blood group tattoo, he was not identified as being on the major war criminal list.[60] He was released at the end of July and obtained false papers under the name "Fritz Ullman", documents he later altered to read "Fritz Hollmann".[61]

After several months on the run, including a trip to the Soviet-occupied area to recover his Auschwitz records, Mengele found work near Rosenheim as a farmhand.[62] Worried that his capture would mean a trial and death sentence, he fled Germany on 17 April 1949.[63][64] Assisted by a network of former SS members, Mengele traveled to Genoa, where he obtained a passport under the alias "Helmut Gregor" from the International Committee of the Red Cross. He sailed to Argentina in July.[65] His wife refused to accompany him, and they divorced in 1954.[66]

17.5   In South America

In Buenos Aires, Argentina, Mengele worked as a carpenter while residing in a boarding house in the suburb of Vicente Lopcz.[67] After a few weeks he moved to the house of a Nazi sympathiser in the more affluent neighborhood of Florida, Buenos Aires. He next worked as a salesman for his family's farm equipment company, and beginning in 1951 he made frequent trips to Paraguay as sales representative for that region.[68] An apartment in the center of Buenos Aires became his residence in 1953, the same year he used family funds to buy a part interest in a carpentry concern. In 1954 he rented a house in the suburb of Olivos.[69] Files released by the Argentine government in 1992 indicate that Mengele may have practiced medicine without a license, including performing abortions, while living in Buenos Aires.[70]

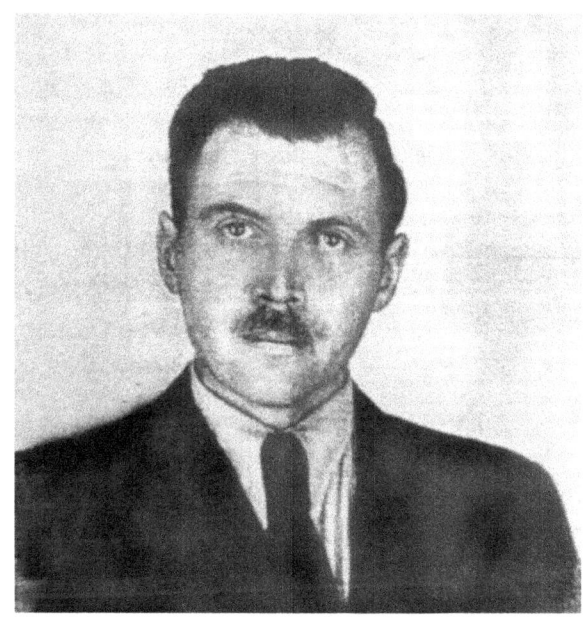

Photo from Mengele's Argentine identification document (1956)

After obtaining a copy of his birth certificate through the West German embassy in 1956, Mengele was issued an Argentine foreign residence permit under his real name. He used this document to obtain a West German passport, also under his real name, and embarked for a visit to Europe.[71][72] He met up in Switzerland for a ski holiday with his son Rolf (who was told Mengele was his "Uncle Fritz"[73]) and his widowed sister-in-law Martha, and spent a week in his home town of Günzburg.[74][75] Upon his return to Argentina in September, Mengele began living under his real name. Martha and her son Karl Heinz followed about a month later, and the three took up residence together. The couple married while on holiday in Uruguay in 1958 and bought a house in Buenos Aires.[71][76] Business interests now included part ownership of Fadro Farm, a pharmaceutical company.[74] Along with several other doctors, Mengele was questioned and released in 1958 under suspicion of practicing medicine without a license after a teenage girl died following an abortion. Worried that the publicity would lead to his Nazi background and wartime activities being discovered, he took an extended business trip to Paraguay and was granted citizenship under the name José Mengele in 1959.[77] He returned to Buenos Aires several times to wrap up his business affairs and visit his family. Martha and Karl Heinz lived in a boarding house in the city until December 1960, when they returned to Germany.[78]

Mengele's name was mentioned several times during the Nuremberg trials, but Allied forces were convinced that he was dead.[79] Irene and the family in Günzburg also said that he was dead.[80] Working in West Germany, Nazi hunters Simon Wiesenthal and Hermann Langbein collected information from witnesses as to Mengele's wartime activities. In a search of the public records, Langbein found Mengele's divorce papers listing an address in Buenos Aires. He and Wiesenthal pressured West German authorities into drawing up an arrest warrant on 5 June 1959, and starting extradition proceedings.[81][82] Initially Argentina turned down the request, because the fugitive was no longer living at the address given on the documents. By the time extradition was approved on 30 June 1960, Mengele had already fled to Paraguay, where he was living on a farm near the Argentine border.[83]

17.5.1   Efforts by the Mossad

In May 1960, Isser Harel, director of the Mossad (the Israeli intelligence agency), personally led the successful effort to capture Adolf Eichmann in Buenos Aires. He hoped to track down Mengele as well so he too could be brought to trial in Israel.[84] Under interrogation, Eichmann provided the address of a boarding house that had been used as a safe house for Nazi fugitives. Surveillance of the house did not reveal Mengele or any members of his family, and the neighborhood postman said that although Mengele had recently been receiving letters there under his real name, he had since relocated, leaving no forwarding address. Harel's inquiries at a machine shop where Mengele had been part owner did not turn up any leads either, so he had to give up.[85]

In spite of having provided Mengele with legal documents in his real name in 1956, thus enabling him to regularize his residency in Argentina, West Germany offered a reward for his capture. Ongoing newspaper coverage of his wartime activities (accompanied by photographs of the fugitive) led Mengele to relocate again in 1960. Former bomber pilot Hans-Ulrich Rudel put him in touch with the Nazi sup-

porter Wolfgang Gerhard, who helped Mengele get across the border into Brazil.[78][86] He stayed with Gerhard on his farm near São Paulo until more permanent accommodations were found with Hungarian expatriates Geza and Gitta Stammer. Helped by an investment from Mengele, the couple bought a farm in Nova Europa, and Mengele was given the job of manager. In 1962 the three bought a coffee and cattle farm in Serra Negra, with Mengele owning a half interest.[87] Initially, Gerhard told the couple that Mengele's name was "Peter Hochbichler", but they discovered his true identity in 1963. Gerhard convinced them not to report Mengele's location to the authorities, saying they could themselves get in trouble for harboring the fugitive.[88] West Germany, tipped off to the possibility that Mengele had relocated there, widened its extradition request to include Brazil in February 1961.[89]

Meanwhile, Zvi Aharoni, one of the Mossad agents who had been involved in the Eichmann capture, was placed in charge of a team of agents tasked with locating Mengele and bringing him to trial in Israel. Inquiries in Paraguay gave no clues as to his whereabouts, and they were unable to intercept any correspondence between Mengele and his wife Martha, then living in Italy. Agents following Rudel's movements did not produce any leads.[90] Aharoni and his team followed Gerhard to a rural area near São Paulo, where they located a European man believed to be Mengele.[91] Aharoni reported his findings to Harel, but the logistics of staging a capture, budgetary constraints, and the need to focus on the nation's deteriorating relationship with Egypt led the Mossad chief to call a halt to the operation in 1962.[92]

17.5.2   Later life and death

Mengele and the Stammers bought a house on a farm in Caieiras in 1969, with Mengele as half owner.[93] When Wolfgang Gerhard returned to Germany in 1971 to seek medical treatment for his seriously ill wife and son, he gave his identity card to Mengele.[94] The Stammers had a falling out with Mengele in late 1974 and bought a house in São Paulo; Mengele was not invited.[lower-alpha 2] The Stammers bought a bungalow in Eldorado, São Paulo, which they rented out to Mengele.[97] Rolf, who had not seen his father since the ski holiday in 1956, visited him there in 1977 and found an unrepentant Nazi who claimed he had never personally harmed anyone and had only done his duty.[98]

Mengele's health had been steadily deteriorating since 1972, and he had a stroke in 1976.[99] He had high blood pressure and an ear infection that had an impact on his balance. While visiting his friends Wolfram and Liselotte Bossert in the coastal resort of Bertioga on 7 February 1979, he suffered another stroke while swimming and drowned.[100] Mengele was buried in Embu das Artes under the name "Wolfgang Gerhard", whose identification card he had been using since 1971.[101]

Other pseudonyms used by Mengele included Dr. Fausto Rindón and S. Josi Alvers Aspiazu.[102]

17.6 Exhumation

Meanwhile, Mengele sightings were reported all over the world. Wiesenthal claimed to have information that placed Mengele on the Greek island of Kythnos in 1960,[103] Cairo in 1961,[104] in Spain in 1971,[105] and in Paraguay in 1978, eighteen years after he had left.[106] He insisted as late as 1985—six years after Mengele's death—that he was still alive, in 1982 offering a reward of $100,000 for his capture.[107] Worldwide interest in the case was raised by a mock trial held in Jerusalem in February 1985 featuring the testimony of over a hundred victims of Mengele's experiments. Shortly afterwards, the governments of West Germany, Israel, and the United States launched a coordinated effort to determine Mengele's whereabouts. Rewards for his capture were offered by the Israeli and West German governments, *The Washington Times*, and the Simon Wiesenthal Center.[108]

On 31 May 1985, acting on a tip received by the West German prosecutor's office, police raided the house of Hans Sedlmeier, a lifelong friend of Mengele and sales manager of the family firm in Günzburg.[109] They found a coded address book and copies of letters to and from Mengele. Among the papers was a letter from Bossert notifying Sedlmeier of Mengele's death.[110] German authorities notified the police in São Paulo, who contacted the Bosserts. Under interrogation, they revealed the location of the grave.[111] The remains were exhumed on 6 June 1985, and extensive forensic examination confirmed with a high degree of probability that the body was Mengele's.[112] Rolf Mengele issued a statement on 10 June admitting the body was his father's. He said the news of his father's death had been kept quiet to protect the people who had sheltered his father for so many years.[113] In 1992, DNA testing verified Mengele's identity.[114] The family refused to have the remains repatriated to Germany, and they remain stored at the São Paulo Institute for Forensic Medicine.[115]

17.7 Legacy

Mengele's life was the inspiration for a novel and movie titled *The Boys from Brazil* (1978), where a fictional Mengele (portrayed by Gregory Peck[116]) produces clones of Hitler in a clinic in Brazil. [117] In 2007, the United States Holocaust Memorial Museum received as a donation the Höcker

Album, an album of photographs of Auschwitz staff taken by Karl-Friedrich Höcker. Eight of the photographs include Mengele.[118]

In February 2010, a 180-page volume of Mengele's diary sold at auction for an undisclosed sum to the grandson of a Holocaust survivor. The unidentified previous owner, who acquired the journals in Brazil, was reported to be close to the Mengele family. A Holocaust survivors' organization described the sale as "a cynical act of exploitation aimed at profiting from the writings of one of the most heinous Nazi criminals."[119] Rabbi Marvin Hier of the Simon Wiesenthal Center was glad to see the diary fall into Jewish hands. "At a time when Ahmadinejad's Iran regularly denies the Holocaust and anti-Semitism and hatred of Jews is back in vogue, this acquisition is especially significant," he said.[120] In 2011, a further 31 volumes of Mengele's diaries were sold—again amidst protests—by the same auction house to an undisclosed collector of World War II memorabilia for $245,000.[121]

17.8 Summary of SS career

- SS number: 317,885

- Nazi Party number: 5,574,974

- Primary positions: *WVHA*, Medical Physician (Auschwitz Concentration Camp)

- *Waffen-SS* Service:

  - Medical Staff Officer, *Waffen-SS* Medical Inspectorate (1940)

  - Medical Officer, Pioneer Battalion No. 5, 5th SS Panzer Division Wiking (1941–1943)

  - Medical Officer, Battalion "Ost", 3rd SS Division Totenkopf (1943)

Dates of rank

Awards

- Iron Cross (First and Second Class)

- War Merit Cross (Second Class with Swords)

- Eastern Front Medal

- Wound Badge (Black)

- Social Welfare Decoration

- German Sports Badge (Bronze)

- Honour Chevron for the Old Guard[lower-alpha 4]

17.9 Journal articles

- *Racial-Morphological Examinations of the Anterior Portion of the Lower Jaw in Four Racial Groups.* This dissertation, completed in 1935 and first published in 1937, earned him a PhD in anthropology from Munich University. In this work Mengele sought to demonstrate that there were structural differences in the lower jaws of individuals from different ethnic groups, and that racial distinctions could be made based on these differences.[7][123]

- *Genealogical Studies in the Cases of Cleft Lip-Jaw-Palate* (1938), his medical dissertation, earned him a doctorate in medicine from Frankfurt University. Studying the influence of genetics as a factor in the occurrence of this deformity, Mengele conducted research on families who exhibited these traits in multiple generations. The work also included notes on other abnormalities found in these family lines.[7][124]

- *Hereditary Transmission of Fistulae Auris.* This journal article, published in *Der Erbarzt* (The Genetic Physician), focuses on fistula auris (an abnormal fissure on the external ear) as a hereditary trait. Mengele noted that individuals who have this trait also tend to have a dimple on their chin.[13]

17.10 See also

- Nazi eugenics

- Shirō Ishii, director of Imperial Japan's Unit 731 facility in World War II, involved in illegal human experimentation

17.11 Notes

[1] Of the Hungarians who arrived in mid-1944, 85 percent were killed immediately.[28]

[2] Based on entries in Mengele's journals and interviews with his friends, historians such as Gerald Posner and Gerald Astor believe he had a sexual relationship with Gitta Stammer.[95][96]

[3] Mengele's enlisted service is mentioned on only a single document of his official SS file. His entry date into the SS is stated to have occurred in early 1938, and by the date of his commissioning in 1940, Mengele was serving as an SS-First Sergeant in the *Waffen-SS* Reserve.[122]

[4] Mengele's SS service record indicates this decoration, even though he was not a Nazi Party or SS member prior to

1933, which was a primary requirement for the Old Guard Chevron.[122]

17.12 References

[1] Levy 2006, p. 242.

[2] Kubica 1998, p. 320.

[3] Astor 1985, p. 102.

[4] Astor 1985, p. 12.

[5] Posner & Ware 1986, pp. 4–5.

[6] Posner & Ware 1986, pp. 6–7.

[7] Kubica 1998, p. 318.

[8] Kershaw 2008, p. 81.

[9] Posner & Ware 1986, pp. 8, 10.

[10] Weindling 2002, p. 53.

[11] Allison 2011, p. 52.

[12] Levy 2006, p. 234 (footnote).

[13] Lifton 1986, p. 340.

[14] Posner & Ware 1986, p. 11.

[15] Posner & Ware 1986, p. 54.

[16] Evans 2008, p. 7.

[17] Longerich 2010, p. 132.

[18] Posner & Ware 1986, p. 16.

[19] Kubica 1998, pp. 318–319.

[20] Kubica 1998, p. 319.

[21] Posner & Ware 1986, pp. 16–18.

[22] Astor 1985, p. 27.

[23] Allison 2011, p. 53.

[24] Steinbacher 2005, p. 94.

[25] Longerich 2010, pp. 282–283.

[26] Steinbacher 2005, pp. 104–105.

[27] Rees 2005, p. 100.

[28] Steinbacher 2005, p. 109.

[29] Levy 2006, pp. 235–237.

[30] Astor 1985, p. 80.

[31] Levy 2006, pp. 248–249.

[32] Posner & Ware 1986, p. 29.

[33] Posner & Ware 1986, p. 27.

[34] Lifton 1985.

[35] Astor 1985, p. 78.

[36] Piper 1998, pp. 170, 172.

[37] Kubica 1998, pp. 328–329.

[38] Posner & Ware 1986, p. 33.

[39] Posner & Ware 1986, pp. 33–34.

[40] Steinbacher 2005, p. 114.

[41] Lifton 1986, pp. 358–359.

[42] Nyiszli 2011, p. 57.

[43] Kubica 1998, pp. 320–321.

[44] Lagnado & Dekel 1991, p. 9.

[45] Lifton 1986, p. 341.

[46] Lifton 1986, pp. 376–377.

[47] Posner & Ware 1986, p. 48.

[48] Lifton 1985, p. 337.

[49] Lifton 1986, p. 350.

[50] Posner & Ware 1986, p. 37.

[51] Lifton 1986, p. 351.

[52] Lifton 1986, pp. 347, 353.

[53] Lifton 1986, p. 362.

[54] Lifton 1986, p. 360.

[55] Brozan 1982.

[56] Mozes-Kor 1992, p. 57.

[57] Levy 2006, p. 255.

[58] Posner & Ware 1986, p. 57.

[59] Steinbacher 2005, p. 128.

[60] Posner & Ware 1986, p. 63.

[61] Posner & Ware 1986, pp. 63, 68.

[62] Posner & Ware 1986, pp. 68, 88.

[63] Posner & Ware 1986, p. 87.

[64] Levy 2006, p. 263.

[65] Levy 2006, p. 264–265.

[66] Posner & Ware 1986, pp. 88,108.

[67] Posner & Ware 1986, p. 95.

[68] Posner & Ware 1986, pp. 104–105.

[69] Posner & Ware 1986, pp. 107–108.

[70] Nash 1992.

[71] Levy 2006, p. 267.

[72] Astor 1985, p. 166.

[73] Posner & Ware 1986, p. 2.

[74] Astor 1985, p. 167.

[75] Posner & Ware 1986, p. 111.

[76] Posner & Ware 1986, p. 112.

[77] Levy 2006, pp. 269–270.

[78] Levy 2006, p. 273.

[79] Posner & Ware 1986, pp. 76, 82.

[80] Levy 2006, p. 261.

[81] Levy 2006, p. 271.

[82] Posner & Ware 1986, p. 121.

[83] Levy 2006, pp. 269–270, 272.

[84] Posner & Ware 1986, p. 139.

[85] Posner & Ware 1986, pp. 142–143.

[86] Posner & Ware 1986, p. 162.

[87] Levy 2006, pp. 279–281.

[88] Levy 2006, pp. 280, 282.

[89] Posner & Ware 1986, p. 168.

[90] Posner & Ware 1986, pp. 166–167.

[91] Posner & Ware 1986, pp. 184–186.

[92] Posner & Ware 1986, pp. 184, 187–188.

[93] Posner & Ware 1986, p. 223.

[94] Levy 2006, p. 289.

[95] Posner & Ware 1986, pp. 178–179.

[96] Astor 1985, p. 224.

[97] Levy 2006, pp. 242–243.

[98] Posner & Ware 1986, pp. 2, 279.

[99] Levy 2006, pp. 289, 291.

[100] Levy 2006, pp. 294–295.

[101] Blumenthal 1985, p. 1.

[102] Zentner & Bedürftig 1991, p. 586.

[103] Segev 2010, p. 167.

[104] Walters 2009, p. 317.

[105] Walters 2009, p. 370.

[106] Levy 2006, p. 296.

[107] Levy 2006, pp. 297, 301.

[108] Posner & Ware 1986, pp. 306–308.

[109] Posner & Ware 1986, pp. 89, 313.

[110] Levy 2006, p. 302.

[111] Posner & Ware 1986, pp. 315, 317.

[112] Posner & Ware 1986, pp. 319–321.

[113] Posner & Ware 1986, p. 322.

[114] Saad 2005.

[115] Simons 1988.

[116] Turner 2003.

[117] Levy 2006, p. 287.

[118] USHMM website.

[119] Oster 2010.

[120] Hier 2010.

[121] Aderet 2011.

[122] SS service record, NARA.

[123] Lifton 1986, p. 339.

[124] Lifton 1986, pp. 339–340.

17.13   Sources

- Aderet, Ofer (22 July 2011). "Ultra-Orthodox man buys diaries of Nazi doctor Mengele for $245,000". *Haaretz*. Retrieved 2 February 2014.

- Allison, Kirk C. (2011). "Eugenics, race hygiene, and the Holocaust: Antecedents and consolidations". In Friedman, Jonathan C. *Routledge History of the Holocaust*. Milton Park; New York: Taylor & Francis. pp. 45–58. ISBN 978-0-415-77956-2.

- Astor, Gerald (1985). *Last Nazi: Life and Times of Dr Joseph Mengele*. New York: Donald I. Fine. ISBN 0-917657-46-2.

- Blumenthal, Ralph (22 July 1985). "Scientists Decide Brazil Skeleton Is Josef Mengele". *New York Times* (Arthur Ochs Sulzberger, Jr.). Retrieved 1 February 2014.

- Brozan, Nadine (15 November 1982). "Out of Death, a Zest for Life". *The New York Times*.

- Evans, Richard J. (2008). *The Third Reich at War*. New York: Penguin. ISBN 978-0-14-311671-4.

- Hier, Marvin (2010). "Wiesenthal Center Praises Acquisition of Mengele's Diary". Simpn Wiesenthal Center. Retrieved 2 February 2014.

- Kershaw, Ian (2008). *Hitler: A Biography*. New York: W. W. Norton & Company. ISBN 978-0-393-06757-6.

- Kubica, Helena (1998) [1994]. "The Crimes of Josef Mengele". In Gutman, Yisrael; Berenbaum, Michael. *Anatomy of the Auschwitz Death Camp*. Bloomington, Indiana: Indiana University Press. pp. 317–337. ISBN 978-0-253-20884-2.

- Lagnado, Lucette Matalon; Dekel, Sheila Cohn (1991). *Children of the Flames: Dr Josef Mengele and the Untold Story of the Twins of Auschwitz*. New York: William Morrow. ISBN 0-688-09695-6.

- Levy, Alan (2006) [1993]. *Nazi Hunter: The Wiesenthal File* (Revised 2002 ed.). London: Constable & Robinson. ISBN 978-1-84119-607-7.

- Lifton, Robert Jay (21 July 1985). "What Made This Man? Mengele". *The New York Times*. Retrieved 11 January 2014.

- Lifton, Robert Jay (1986). *The Nazi Doctors: Medical Killing and the Psychology of Genocide*. New York: Basic Books. ISBN 978-0-465-04905-9.

- Longerich, Peter (2010). *Holocaust: The Nazi Persecution and Murder of the Jews*. Oxford; New York: Oxford University Press. ISBN 978-0-19-280436-5.

- Mozes-Kor, Eva (1992). "Mengele Twins and Human Experimentation: A Personal Account". In Annas, George J.; Grodin, Michael A. *The Nazi Doctors and the Nuremberg Code: Human Rights in Human Experimentation*. New York: Oxford University Press. pp. 53–59. ISBN 978-0-19-510106-5.

- Nash, Nathaniel C. (11 February 1992). "Mengele an Abortionist, Argentine Files Suggest". *The New York Times*. Retrieved 31 August 2014.

- Nyiszli, Miklós (2011) [1960]. *Auschwitz: A Doctor's Eyewitness Account*. New York: Arcade Publishing. ISBN 978-1-61145-011-8.

- Oster, Marcy (3 February 2010). "Survivor's grandson buys Mengele diary". Jewish Telegraphic Agency. Retrieved 2 February 2014.

- Piper, Franciszek (1998) [1994]. "Gas Chambers and Crematoria". In Gutman, Yisrael; Berenbaum, Michael. *Anatomy of the Auschwitz Death Camp*. Bloomington, Indiana: Indiana University Press. pp. 157–182. ISBN 978-0-253-20884-2.

- Posner, Gerald L.; Ware, John (1986). *Mengele: The Complete Story*. New York: McGraw-Hill. ISBN 0-07-050598-5.

- Rees, Laurence (2005). *Auschwitz: A New History*. New York: Public Affairs. ISBN 1-58648-303-X.

- Saad, Rana (1 April 2005). "Discovery, development, and current applications of DNA identity testing". *Baylor University Medical Center Proceedings* **18** (2): 130–133. PMC 1200713. PMID 16200161.

- Segev, Tom (2010). *Simon Wiesenthal: The Life and Legends*. New York: Doubleday. ISBN 978-0-385-51946-5.

- Simons, Marlise (17 March 1988). "Remains of Mengele Rest Uneasily in Brazil". *The New York Times*. Retrieved 2 February 2014.

- "SS service record of Josef Mengele". College Park, Maryland: National Archives and Records Administration.

- Steinbacher, Sybille (2005) [2004]. *Auschwitz: A History*. Munich: Verlag C. H. Beck. ISBN 0-06-082581-2.

- "The Album". United States Holocaust Memorial Museum. 2007. Retrieved 2 February 2014.

- Turner, Adrian (14 June 2003). "Gregory Peck: Elder statesman of the screen who stood for nobility, honour and decency". *The Independent*. Retrieved 1 September 2015.

- Walters, Guy (2009). *Hunting Evil: The Nazi War Criminals Who Escaped and the Quest to Bring Them to Justice*. New York: Broadway Books. ISBN 978-0-7679-2873-1.

- Weindling, Paul (2002). "The Ethical Legacy of Nazi Medical War Crimes: Origins, Human Experiments, and International Justice". In Burley, Justine; Harris, John. *A Companion to Genethics*. Blackwell Companions to Philosophy. Malden, MA; Oxford: Blackwell. pp. 53–69. doi:10.1002/9780470756423.ch5. ISBN 0-631-20698-1.

- Zentner, Christian; Bedürftig, Friedemann (1991). *The Encyclopedia of the Third Reich*. New York: Macmillan. ISBN 0-02-897502-2.

17.14 Further reading

- Harel, Isser (1975). *The House on Garibaldi Street: the First Full Account of the Capture of Adolf Eichmann*. New York: Viking Press. ISBN 0-670-38028-8.

- Levin, Ira (1991). *The Boys from Brazil*. London: Bantam. ISBN 0-553-29004-5.

- Lieberman, Herbert A. (1978). *The Climate of Hell*. New York: Simon and Schuster. ISBN 0-671-82236-5.

17.15 External links

- Breitman, Richard (April 2001). "Historical Analysis of 20 Name Files from CIA Records". US National Archives.

- Office of Special Investigations, Criminal Division (October 1992). "In the Matter of Josef Mengele: A Report to the Attorney General of the United States" (PDF). United States Department of Justice.

- Papanayotou, Vivi (18 September 2005). "Skeletons in the Closet of German Science". Deutsche Welle.

- Posner, Gerald; Ware, John (18 May 1986). "How Nazi war criminal Josef Mengele cheated justice for 34 years". *Chicago Tribune Magazine*.

Chapter 18

Otfrid Mittmann

Otfrid Mittmann (born 27 Dec 1908 in Ruda Śląska;[1][2] probably killed in WWII)[2] was a German mathematician. Starting in 1927, he studied mathematics and natural sciences in Göttingen and Leipzig, and got his Ph.D. in Apr 1935.[2] He joined the Nazi movement in Oct 1929.[3] and published on statistical aspects of Nazi eugenics.

18.1 Publications

- Mittmann, O. (1935). *Mathematisch-statistische Untersuchungen zur Erforschung fließender Merkmale* (Ph.D. thesis). Univ. Göttingen.

- Mittmann, Otfrid (1936). *Über die Schnelligkeit der relativen Vermehrung vorteilhafter Mutationen*. Göttingen: Vandenhoeck & Ruprecht.

- Otfrid Mittmann (May 1936). "Zur Austilgung einer vererbbaren Eigenschaft bei Merkmalen mit übergreifenden Erscheinungformen (Fall des einpaarigen Erbgangs)". *Deutsche Mathematik* **1** (2): 149—155.

- Otfrid Mittmann (Apr 1937). "Die Erfolgsaussichten von Auslesemaßnahmen im Kampf gegen die Erbkrankheiten". *Deutsche Mathematik* **2** (1): 32—55. Man pflegt leider mit einem derartig unsauberen Verfahren zu arbeiten, wenn es sich darum handelt, ein Urteil über den Wert des deutschen Gesetzes zur Verhütung erbkranken Nachwuchses in die Welt zu setzen. Es soll im folgenden kurz gezeigt werden, wie die Dinge liegen und welche Extremfälle man sich auszusuchen pflegt, um ein möglichst ungünstiges Urteil über den Wert der deutschen Auslesemaßnahmen zu gewinnen. *(Unfortunately, one uses to work with such an unsound approach when a judgement about the German Law for the Prevention of Hereditarily Diseased Offspring is to be created. In the following, it shall be shown how things are and which extremal cases one uses to pick out to obtain an as unfavorable judgement as possible about the value of the German selection measures.)*

- Otfrid Mittmann (Jan 1938). "Über die Schnelligkeit der Ausmerze von Erbkrankheiten durch Sterilisation". *Deutsche Mathematik* **2** (6): 709—721.

- Mittmann, Otfrid (1940). *Erbbiologische Fragen in mathematischer Behandlung*. Berlin: de Gruyter.

- Otfrid Mittmann (Dec 1940). "Theoretische Erbprognose und Gattenwahl". *Deutsche Mathematik* **5** (4): 328—337.

- Otfrid Mittmann (May 1941). "Funktionale Zusammenhänge zwischen Zygotenwahrscheinlichkeiten". *Deutsche Mathematik* **5** (6): 563—570.

18.2 References

[1] Record and German National Library

[2] Volkmar Weiss (1982). "Klassischer und probabilistischer Mendelismus: Ein wissenschaftsgeschichtlicher Beitrag zur Latenz wissenschaftlicher Ideen". *Biologisches Zentralblatt* **101**: 597—607.

[3] Vita (p.10) at German Mathematical Society

18.3 External links

- Otfrid Mittmann at the Mathematics Genealogy Project

Chapter 19

Alfred Ploetz

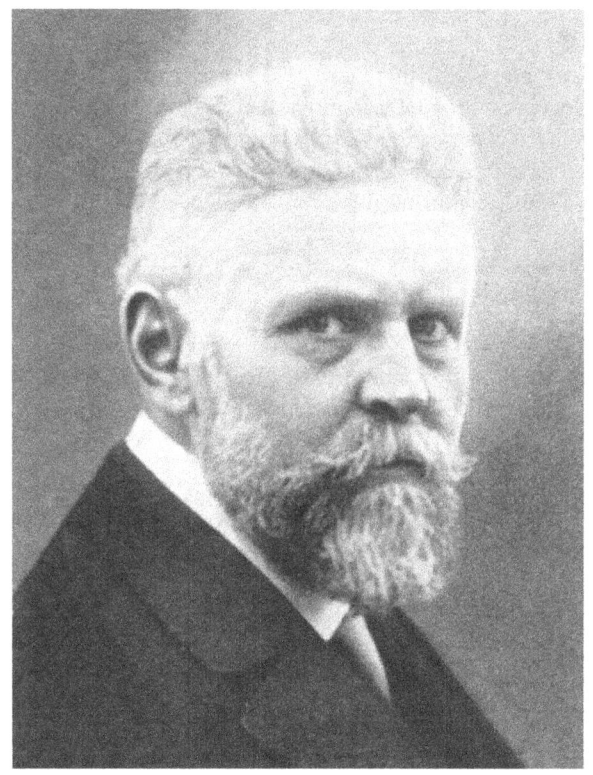

Alfred Ploetz

Alfred Ploetz (August 22, 1860 – March 20, 1940) was a German physician, biologist, eugenicist known for coining the term racial hygiene (*Rassenhygiene*)[1] and promoting the concept in Germany. *Rassenhygiene* is a form of eugenics.

19.1 Life and career

Alfred Ploetz was born in Swinemünde, Germany (now Świnoujście, Poland) and he grew up and attended school in Breslau (now Wrocław). At this time he began his friendship with Carl Hauptmann, brother of the famous author Gerhart Hauptmann. In 1879 he founded a secret racist youth society. In Gerhart Hauptmann's Drama "Vor Sonnenaufgang" (Before Sunrise) which was first performed on October 20, 1889 in Berlin, the key figure of the journalist Loth is based on Ploetz.

After school Ploetz at first studied political economy in Breslau. There he joined the "Freie wissenschaftliche Vereinigung" (free scientific union). Among his friends were – besides his brother – his former school friend Ferdinand Simon (later son-in-law of August Bebel), the brothers Carl and Gerhart Hauptmann, Heinrich Laux, and Charles Proteus Steinmetz.

This circle enthusiastically read the works of Ernst Haeckel and Charles Darwin. Carl Hauptmann was a student of Ernst Haeckel, and Gerhart Hauptmann and Ploetz attended some of his lectures. The group expanded and developed a plan of founding a colony in one of the pacific states and established itself as the "Pacific association". They planned a "community on friendly, socialist and maybe also pan-Germanic basis". In consequence of the prosecution of socialistically minded persons in application of Otto von Bismarck's anti-socialist laws (1878–1890), in 1883 Ploetz fled to Zurich, where he continued to study political economy with Julius Platter (1844–1923). In his memoirs Ploetz states as an important reason for his choice of Zurich that in his studies in Breslau socialist theories were only incidentally mentioned.

After living for a half a year in the United States, Ploetz returned to Zurich and began to study medicine. In 1886 he fell in love with a fellow student Agnes Bluhm despite being involved with Pauline Rüdin. They decided to get married early in 1887. Ploetz was also seeing an American named Mary Sherwood who was studying hypnotism. In 1890 Ploetz became medical doctor and married his former girlfriend Pauline, though the two never had children. Bluhm however kept Ploetz as a close friend throughout her life and they both shared similar views on racial purity and the benefits of eugenics.[2] Ploetz and his wife lived in the US for four years, and divorced in 1898. Ploetz later married Anita Nordenholz. This marriage produced three children: Ulrich (called Uli), Cordelia (called Deda) and Wilfrid (called Fridl, 1912–2013).[3]

Ploetz first proposed the theory of racial hygiene (race-based eugenics) in his "Racial Hygiene Basics" (*Grundlinien einer Rassenhygiene*) in 1895. In 1904 Ploetz founded the periodical "Archiv für Rassen-und Gesellschaftsbiologie" with Fritz Lenz as chief editor, and in 1905 the German Society for Racial Hygiene (De Berliner Gesellschaft fur Rassenhygiene) [4] with 31 members. page [5] In 1907 the society became the "International Society for Racial Hygiene".[6] In 1930 he became an honorary doctor of the University of Munich.

Ploetz was a supporter of the Nazi Party, which took power in 1933. Ploetz wrote in April 1933 that he believed Hitler would bring racial hygiene from its previous marginality into the mainstream.

In 1933 Reich Interior Minister Wilhelm Frick established an "expert advisory committee for population and racial policy," which included Ploetz, Fritz Lenz, Ernst Rüdin and Hans F.K. Günther. This expert advisory committee had the task of advising the Nazis on the implementation and enforcement of legislation regarding racial and eugenic issues.[7] In 1936, Hitler appointed Ploetz to a professorship.

In 1937 he joined the Nazi party.[8]

He died at the age of 79 and is buried at his home in Herrsching on the Ammersee in Bavaria. After his death, Otmar Freiherr von Verschuer praised his "inner sympathy and enthusiasm [with] the National Socialist Movement".[9] Ernst Rüdin, also a committed National Socialist, praised Ploetz two years before as a man "by his meritorious services has helped to set up our Nazi ideology."[10]

19.2 Theories

In his book *The efficiency of our race and the protection of the weak* (1895) he described a society in which eugenic ideas were applied. Society would examine the moral and intellectual capacity of citizens to decide on marriage and the permitted number of children. It may also include a prohibition on reproduction. Disabled children are aborted, the sick and weak, twins and children whose parents Ploetz considers too old or young, are "eliminated".

Along with many other eugenicists in Europe and America, Ploetz believed in the superiority of the Nordic race. His writings were a major influence on Nazi ideology. His opinion of the Jewish Question changed during the course of his life, but his view and the doctrine of the NSDAP were in accord by the time the party came to power in 1933.

In his early writings Ploetz credited Jews as the second highest cultural race after Europeans.[11] He identified no sub-

stantial difference in "racial character" between Aryans and Jews, arguing that the mental abilities of Jews and their role in the development of human culture made them indispensable to the "process of racial mix" which would enhance humanity.

> The high aptitude of the Jews and their outstanding role in the progress of mankind considering men like Jesus, Spinoza, Marx has to be kindly acknowledged without hesitation... All this Antisemitism is a flop which will vanish slowly in the light of scientific knowledge and a humane democracy".[12]

Later he revised this view. He stressed that the distinctiveness of Jews indicated that their mental characteristics would adversely affect Aryans by introducing individualism and lack of love for the military and the nation. He favored the global dominance of the Aryan race.[13]

19.3 Bibliography

- (Alfred Hoche, Alfred Ploetz, Alfred Vierkandt, Carl Hans Heinze Sennhenn) German Eugenicists: **ISBN9781230541914** [14]

- (Alfred J Ploetz) Die Tüchtigkeit unsrer Rasse und der Schutz der Schwachen **ISBN1103490796** [15]

- (Alfred J Ploetz) Archiv für Rassen- und Gesellschafts-Biologie, einschliesslich Rassen- und Gesellschafts-Hygiene 1908, Fuenfter Jahrgang **ISBN117441166X** [16]

19.4 See also

- Eugen Fischer

- Karl Binding

- Ernst Rudin

- Racial hygiene

- Eugenics

19.5 References

[1] Bashford, Alison; Levine, Phillipa, eds. (2010). "Eugenics and the Modern World". *The Oxford Handbook of the History of Eugenics*. Oxford University Press. p. 15. ISBN 978-0199945054. Retrieved 6 August 2015.

[2] Weindling, Paul (1993). *Health, race, and German politics between national unification and Nazism, 1870-1945* (1st pbk. ed.). Cambridge: Cambridge University Press. p. 74. ISBN 052142397X.

[3] "Anzeige von Wilfrid Ploetz - trauer.merkur.de". *merkur-online.de*.

[4] https://archive.org/details/ MystiekAntisemitismeWaarSprookjesEnWetenschapElkaarOntmoeten

[5] Schafft, Gretchen Engle: "From Racism to Genocide: Anthropology in the Third Reich". University of Illinois Press. 2004. Pg. 42.

[6] Atkins, Stephen E. (2009). *Holocaust Denial as an International Movement*. Greenwood Press. p. 24. ISBN 978-0313345388.

[7] Anahid S. Rickman: "Rassenpflege im völkischen Staat", Vom Verhältnis der Rassenhygiene zur nationalsozialistischen Politik. Dissertation Bonn 2002, Online einsehbar unter [3], p. 331

[8] Federal Archives Act Party Zehlendorf.

[9] Otmar von Verschuer, "Alfred Ploetz," in The Erbarzt, Bd 8 p.69-72, 1940, p.71

[10] Ernst Rudin: "Honor of Prof. Dr. Alfred Ploetz," in ARGB, Bd 32 / S.473–474, 1938, p.474

[11] "Wir haben frueher die Juden neben den Westariern als hoechstentwickelte Culturrasse angefuehrt." Ploetz, 137

[12] "Die Tüchtigkeit unserer Rasse und der Schutz der Schwachen", 1893, p. 141, 142. cited by Massimo Ferari Zumbini: The roots of evil. Gründerjahre des Antisemitismus: Von der Bismarckzeit zu Hitler , Vittorio Klostermann, Frankfurt a. M. 2003, ISBN 3-465-03222-5, p.406

[13] Julia Schäfer: "Vermessen – gezeichnet – verlacht Judenbilder in populären Zeitschriften 1918–1933." Campus Verlag, 2005, ISBN 3-593-37745-4, p. 182

[14] https://books.google.be/books?id=q81sngEACAAJ& dq=alfred+ploetz&hl=en&sa=X&ved=0ahUKEwiT_ auamJzKAhUELA8KHYsCB_YQ6AEIJTAB

[15] http://www.amazon.com/T%C3% BCchtigkeit-unsrer-Rasse-Schutz-Schwachen/dp/ 1103490796/ref=sr_1_1?s=books&ie=UTF8&qid= 1452324296&sr=1-1&refinements=p_27%3AAlfred+J. +Ploetz

[16] http://www.amazon.com/ Gesellschafts-Biologie-einschliesslich-Gesellschafts-Hygiene-Fuenfter-Jahrgang/ dp/117441166X/ref=sr_1_6?s=books&ie=UTF8&qid= 1452324296&sr=1-6&refinements=p_27%3AAlfred+J. +Ploetz

19.6 External links

- Works by or about Alfred Ploetz at Internet Archive

Chapter 20

Ernst Rüdin

Ernst Rüdin (April 19, 1874 in St. Gallen – October 22, 1952) was a Swiss-born German psychiatrist, geneticist, eugenicist and Nazi. Rising to prominence under Emil Kraepelin and assuming his directorship at what is now called the Max Planck Institute of Psychiatry in Munich, he has long been scientifically honoured and cited internationally as the pioneer of psychiatric inheritance studies. He also argued for, designed, justified and funded the mass sterilization and clinical killing of adults and children.

20.1   Early career

Commencing in 1893 Rudin studied medicine at universities in several countries, graduating in 1898. In Zurich he worked as assistant to Eugene Bleuler who coined the term 'schizophrenia'. He completed his PhD, then a psychiatric residency at a Berlin prison. From 1907 he worked at the University of Munich as assistant to Emil Kraepelin, the highly influential psychiatrist who had developed the diagnostic split between 'dementia praecox' ('early dementia' - reflecting his pessimistic prognosis - renamed schizophrenia) and 'manic-depressive illness' (including unipolar depression), and who is considered by many to be the father of modern psychiatric classification.[1] Rudin became senior lecturer in 1909 as well as senior physician at the Munich Psychiatric Hospital, succeeding Alois Alzheimer.[2]

Kraepelin and Rudin were both ardent advocates of a theory that the German race was becoming overly 'domesticated' and thus degenerating into higher rates of mental illness and other conditions.[3] Fears of degeneration were somewhat common internationally at the time, but the extent to which Rudin took them may have been unique, and from the very beginning of his career he made continuous efforts to have his research translate into political action. He also repeatedly drew attention to the financial burden of the sick and disabled.[4]

Rüdin developed the concept of "empirical genetic prognosis" of mental disorders. He published influential initial results on the genetics of schizophrenia in 1916.[5]

Rudin's data did not show a high enough risk in siblings for schizophrenia to be due to a simple recessive gene as he and Kraepelin thought, but he put forward a two-recessive-gene theory to try to account for this.[6] This has been attributed to a "mistaken belief" that just one or a small number of gene variations caused such conditions.[7] Nevertheless, Rudin pioneered and refined complex techniques for conducting studies of inheritance, was widely cited in the international literature for decades, and is still regarded as "the father of psychiatric genetics".[8]

Rudin was influenced by his then brother-in-law, and longtime friend and colleague, Alfred Ploetz, who was considered the 'father' of racial hygiene and indeed had coined the term in 1895.[9] This was a form of eugenics, inspired by social darwinism, which had gained some popularity internationally, as would the voluntary or compulsory sterilization of psychiatric patients, initially in America. Rudin campaigned for this early on. At a conference on alcoholism in 1903, he argued for the sterilisation of 'incurable alcoholics', but his proposal was roundly defeated.[9] In 1904 he was appointed co-editor in chief of the newly founded Archive for Racial Hygiene and Social Biology, and in 1905 was among the co-founders of the German Society for Racial Hygiene (which soon became International), along with Ploetz.[10] He published an article of his own in Archives in 1910, in which he argued that medical care for the mentally ill, alcoholics, epileptics and others was a distortion of natural laws of natural selection, and medicine should help to clean the genetic pool.[3]

20.2   Increasing influence

In 1917 a new German Institute for Psychiatric Research was established in Munich (known as the DFA in German; renamed the Max Planck Institute of Psychiatry after WWII), designed and driven forward by Emil Kraepelin. The Institute incorporated a Department of Genealogical and Demographic Studies (known as the GDA in German) - the first in the world specialising in psychiatric genetics - and Rudin was put in charge by overall director Kraepelin. In 1924 the Institute came under the umbrella of the prestigious Kaiser Wilhelm Society. From 1925 Rudin spent three years as full Professor of Psychology at Basel, Switzerland.[10] He returned to the Institute in 1928, with an expanded departmental budget and new building at 2 Kraepelinstrasse, financed primarily by the American Rockefeller Foundation. The institute soon gained an international reputation as leading psychiatric research, including in hereditary genetics. In 1931, a few years after Kraepelin's death, Rudin took over the directorship of the entire Institute as well as remaining head of his department.[4][7][11][12]

Rudin was among the first to attempt to educate the public about the "dangers" of hereditary defectives and the value of the Nordic race as "culture creators".[13] By 1920 his colleague Alfred Hoche published, with lawyer Karl Binding, the influential "Allowing the Destruction of Life Unworthy of Living".[14]

In 1930 Rudin was a leading German representative at the First International Congress for Mental Hygiene, held in Washington, US, arguing for eugenics.[10] In 1932 he became President of the International Federation of Eugenics Organizations. He was in contact with Carlos Blacker of the British Eugenics Society, and sent him a copy of pre-Nazi voluntary sterilization laws enacted in Prussia; a precursor to the Nazi forced sterilization laws that Rudin is said to have already prepared in his desk drawer.[15]

From 1935 to 1945 he was President of the Society of German Neurologists and Psychiatrists (GDNP), later renamed the German Association for Psychiatry and Psychotherapy (DGPPN).[16]

The American Rockefeller Foundation funded numerous international researchers to visit and work at Rudin's psychiatric genetics department, even as late as 1939. These included Eliot Slater and Erik Stromgren, considered the founding fathers of psychiatric genetics in Britain and Scandinavia respectively, as well as Franz Josef Kallmann who became a leading figure in twins research in the US after emigrating in 1936.[4] Kallmann had claimed in 1935 that 'minor anomalies' in otherwise unaffected relatives of schizophrenics should be grounds for compulsory sterilization.

Rudin's research was also supported with manpower and financing from the German National Socialists.

20.3 Nazi expert

In 1933, Ernst Rüdin, Alfred Ploetz, and several other experts on racial hygiene were brought together to form the Expert Committee on Questions of Population and Racial Policy under Reich Interior Minister Wilhelm Frick. The committee's ideas were used as a scientific basis to justify the racial policy of Nazi Germany and its "Law for the Prevention of Hereditarily Diseased Offspring" was passed by the German government on January 1, 1934. Rudin was such an avid proponent that colleagues nicknamed him the "Reichsfuhrer for Sterilization"[2][17]

In a speech to the German Society for *Rassenhygiene* published in 1934, Rudin recalled the early days of trying to alert the public to the special value of the Nordic race and the dangers of defectives. He stated: "The significance of *Rassenhygiene* [racial hygiene] did not become evident to all aware Germans until the political activity of Adolf Hitler and only through his work has our 30-year-long dream of translating *Rassenhygiene* into action finally become a reality." Describing it as a 'duty of honour' for society to help implement the Nazi policies, Rudin declared: "Whoever is not physically or mentally fit must not pass on his defects to his children. The state must take care that only the fit produce children. Conversely, it must be regarded as reprehensible to withhold healthy children from the state."[13]

From early on Rudin had been a 'racial fanatic' for the purity of the 'German people'.[18] However he was also described in 1988 as "not so much a fanatical Nazi as a fanatical geneticist".[19] His ideas for reducing new cases of schizophrenia would prove a total failure, despite between 73% and 100% of the diagnosed being sterilised or killed.[7]

Rudin joined the Nazi party in 1937.[20] In 1939, on his 65th birthday, he was awarded a 'Goethe medal for art and science' handed to him personally by Hitler, who honoured him as the 'pioneer of the racial-hygienic measures of the Third Reich'. In 1944 he received a bronze Nazi eagle medal (Adlerschild des Deutschen Reiches), with Hitler calling him the 'pathfinder in the field of hereditary hygiene'.[10]

In 1942, speaking about 'euthanasia', Rudin emphasised "the value of eliminating young children of clearly inferior quality". He supported and financially aided the work of Julius Duessen at Heidelberg University with Carl Schneider, clinical research which from the beginning involving killing children.[4][17][21][22]

20.4 Post-war

At the end of the war in 1945, Rudin claimed he had only ever engaged in academic science, only ever heard rumours of killings at the nearby insane asylums, and that he hated the Nazis. However, some of his Nazi political activities, scientific justifications, and awards from Hitler were already uncovered in 1945 (as were his lecture handouts praising Nordics and disparaging Jews). Investigative journalist Victor H. Bernstein concluded: "I am sure that Prof. Rudin never so much as killed a fly in his 74 years. I am also sure he is one of the most evil men in Germany." Rudin was stripped of his Swiss citizenship which he had held jointly with German, and two months later was placed under house arrest by the Munich Military Government. However, interned in the US, he was released in 1947 after a 'denazification' trial where he was supported by former colleague Kallmann (a eugenicist himself) and famous quantum physicist Max Planck; his only punishment was a 500-mark fine.[23]

Speculation about the reasons for his early release, despite having been considered as a potential criminal defendant for the Nuremberg trials, include the need to restore confidence and order in the German medical profession; his personal and financial connections to prestigious American and British researchers, funding bodies and others; and the fact that he repeatedly cited American eugenic sterilization initiatives to justify his own as legal (indeed the Nuremberg trials carefully avoided highlighting such links in general). Nevertheless, Rudin has been cited as a more senior and influential architect of Nazi crimes than the physician who was sentenced to death, Karl Brandt, or the infamous Josef Mengele who had attended his lectures and been employed by his Institute.[24]

After Rudin's death in 1952 the funeral eulogy was held by Kurt Pohlisch, a close friend who had been professor of psychiatry at Bonn University, director of the second-largest genetics research institute in Germany, and expert Nazi advisor on Action T4.[25]

Rüdin's connections to the Nazis were a major reason for criticisms of psychiatric genetics in Germany after 1945.[5]

He was survived by his daughter, Edith Zerbin-Rüdin, who became a psychiatric geneticist and eugenicist herself. In 1996 Zerbin-Rudin, along with Kenneth S. Kendler, published a series of articles on his work which were criticised by others for whitewashing his racist and later Nazi ideologies and activities (Elliot S. Gershon also notes that Zerbin-Rudin acted as defender and apologist for her father in private conversation and in a transcribed interview published in 1988).[26][20] Kendler and other leading psychiatric genetic authors have been accused as recently as 2013 of producing revisionist historical accounts of Rudin and his 'Munich School'. Three types of account have been identified: "(A) those who write about German psychiatric genetics in the Nazi period, but either fail to mention Rüdin at all, or cast him in a favorable light; (B) those who acknowledge that Rüdin helped promote eugenic sterilization and/or may have worked with the Nazis, but generally paint a positive picture of Rüdin's research and fail to mention his participation in the "euthanasia" killing program; and (C) those who have written that Rüdin committed and supported un-

speakable atrocities."[27][28]

20.5 Partial bibliography

- Über die klinischen Formen der Gefängnisspsychosen, Diss. Zürich, 1901

- (Hrsg.) Studien über Vererbung und Entstehung geistiger Störungen, 1916-1939

- Psychiatrische Indikation zur Sterilisierung, 1929

- (Einl.) Gesetz zur Verhütung erbkranken Nachwuchses vom 14. Juli 1933, 1934

- (Hrsg.) Erblehre und Rassenhygiene im völkischen Staat, 1934

- Die Bedeutung der Eugenik und Genetik für die Psychische Hygiene. Zeitschrift für psychische Hygiene 3 (1930), S. 133-147

20.6 See also

- T-4 Euthanasia Program

- Ethnic cleansing

- Eugenics

- Nazi doctors (list)

- Racial hygiene

- Werner Heyde

- Werner Villinger

- Alfred Ploetz

20.7 References

[1] Abnormal Psychology and Life: A Dimensional Approach Chris Kearney, Timothy Trull. Cengage Learning, 2014

[2] Science and Inhumanity: The Kaiser-Wilhelm/Max Planck Society William E. Seidelman MD, 2001

[3] Brüne, Martin (1 January 2007). "On human self-domestication, psychiatry, and eugenics". *Philosophy, Ethics, and Humanities in Medicine* **2** (1): 21. doi:10.1186/1747-5341-2-21. PMC 2082022. PMID 17919321.

[4] Man, Medicine, and the State Pg 73-

[5] Matthias M. Weber (1996). "Ernst Rüdin, 1874-1952: A German psychiatrist and geneticist". *American Journal of Medical Genetics* **67** (4): 323–331. doi:10.1002/(SICI)1096-8628(19960726)67:4<323::AID-AJMG2>3.0.CO;2-N. PMID 8837697.

[6] Schizophrenia Irving I. Gottesman, CUP Archive, 30 Jun 1982

[7] Torrey EF, Yolken RH (September 2009). "Psychiatric Genocide: Nazi Attempts to Eradicate Schizophrenia". *Schizophr Bull* **36** (1): 26–32. doi:10.1093/schbul/sbp097. PMC 2800142. PMID 19759092.

[8] Models of Madness: Psychological, Social and Biological Approaches to Psychosis 2013. Eds. John Read, Jacqui Dillon. Pg 35. Citing Steeman (2005) & Straus (2006)

[9] Racial Hygiene: Medicine Under the Nazis, 1988, by Robert Proctor. Pg 96-97

[10] Who's Who in Nazi Germany Robert S. Wistrich, Routledge, 4 Jul 2013

[11] Ernst Klee: *Das Personenlexikon zum Dritten Reich. Wer war was vor und nach 1945.* Fischer Taschenbuch Verlag, Zweite aktualisierte Auflage, Frankfurt am Main 2005, ISBN 978-3-596-16048-8, S. 513.

[12] Psychiatric research and science policy in Germany: the history of the Deutsche Forschungsanstalt fur Psychiatrie (German Institute for Psychiatric Research) in Munich from 1917 to 1945 MM. Weber, 2000

[13] The Science and Politics of Racial Research by William Tucker. University of Illinois Press, 1994. Pg121. Original transcript: E. Rudin, "Aufgaben and Ziele der Deutschen Gesellschaft fur Rassenhygiene," Archiv Fur Rassen- und Gesellschafts- biologie 28 (1934): 228-29

[14] Understanding Mental Health: A Critical Realist Exploration By David Pilgrim

[15] The Eugenics Society, Its Sources and Its Critics in Britain Pauline Mazumdar, Routledge, 20 Dec 2005] Pg207

[16] Psychiatry under National Socialism: Remembrance and Responsibility Frank Schneider, 2011

[17] The Missing Gene Jay Joseph, 2006, pg142-

[18] Ernst Rüdin--a Swiss psychiatrist as the leader of Nazi psychiatry--the final solution as a goal Fortschr Neurol Psychiatr. 1996 Sep;64(9):327-43. (Article in German). Peters UH1.

[19] Ethics and Mental Health: The Patient, Profession and Community Michael Robertson, Garry Walter, preface. Original source psychiatrist Robert Jay Lipton in 1988 book Nazi Doctors.

[20] Elliot S. Gershon (1997). "Letter to the Editor: Ernst Rüdin, a Nazi psychiatrist and geneticist". *American Journal of Medical Genetics* **74** (4): 457–458. doi:10.1002/(SICI)1096-8628(19970725)74:4<457::AID-AJMG23>3.0.CO;2-G. PMID 9259388. (Full text via free trial: https://www.deepdyve.com/lp/wiley/ernst-r-din-a-nazi-psychiatrist-and-geneticist-kzSMkPZPQl)

[21] Medicine and Medical Ethics in Nazi Germany: Origins, Practices, Legacies Chapter by V. Roelcke, Pg106

[22] Program and practice of psychiatric genetics at the German Research Institute of Psychiatry under Ernst Rudin: on the relationship between science, politics and the concept of race before and after 1993 by V. Roelcke, 2002

[23] Genetic Research in Psychiatry and Psychology Under the Microscope Jay Joseph. Pg 33-, 48. Original source: Created Nazi Science of Murder Victor H Berstein, 1945, August 21, PM Daily

[24] From a Race of Masters to a Master Race: 1948 To 1848. A.E. Samaan, 8 Feb 2013.

[25] Baltic Eugenics: Bio-Politics, Race and Nation in Interwar Estonia, Latvia and Lithuania 1918-1940 : Volker Roelcke: 3. Eliot Slater and the Institutionalization of Psychiatric Genetics in the United Kingdom pg312 & note 71 on pg 323

[26] Edith Zerbin-Rüdin, Kenneth S. Kendler (1996). "Ernst Rüdin (1874-1952) and his genealogic-demographic department in Munich (1917-1986): An introduction to their family studies of schizophrenia". *American Journal of Medical Genetics* **67** (4): 332–337. doi:10.1002/(SICI)1096-8628(19960726)67:4<332::AID-AJMG3>3.0.CO;2-O. PMID 8837698.

[27] Ernst Rüdin: Hitler's Racial Hygiene Mastermind. J Hist Biol. 2013 Spring;46(1):1-30. doi: 10.1007/s10739-012-9344-6.

[28] Understanding Mental Health: A Critical Realist Exploration David Pilgrim. Pg 51-

20.8 External links

- History of Mental Health: 1874: Ernst Rüdin By Henk van Setten

- The Simon Wiesenthal Center Multimedia Learning Center Online: Ernst Rudin (nb: page moved)

- International Eugenics

Chapter 21

Carl Schneider

Not to be confused with Kurt Schneider.

Carl Schneider (December 19, 1891 in Gembitz, Kreis Mogilno, Province of Posen – December 11, 1946 in Frankfurt am Main), professor at Heidelberg University, (1933–1945)[1] chairman of its department of Psychiatry,[2] director of its clinic, was a senior researcher for the Action T4 Euthanasia program.

Schneider is said to exemplify the descent of a distinguished academic psychiatrist into the Nazi worldview. Some described him as having shown great empathy in his psychiatric rehabilitation work, and having a great idealism about transforming the 'horror' of psychiatric patients thought to be regressed, isolated and backward. He would sometimes put forward two possible ways of helping a patient - one of them 'work therapy', and the other to sterilize or kill them.[3]

Schneider joined the Nazi Party in 1932. He defined and elaborated the psychological assumptions of Nazi ideology and science. He coined the term *National therapy* for ethnic cleansing: ridding the populace of genetic and blood contaminants threatening the psychological and physical health of the German/Aryan population.[4] He collected the brains of murdered Jews,[2] retarded children, and other victims, for research in his clinic and for instruction. He taught a technique of replacing spinal fluid with air, to get clearer x-rays of the brain.

Schneider, along with Konrad Zucker, helped Heidelberg become one of the two leading training centres for the killing of children for theoretically scientific purposes, which went on at thirty clinics for three years.[5]

After the war, the U.S. occupation authorities barred his reinstatement to the university's medical faculty, even before they learned of his role in the euthanasia program. They later arrested him. Professor Schneider hanged himself in his prison cell (1946) awaiting trial in Frankfurt am Main.[6][7][8]

21.1 References

[1] Shorter, Edward (2005). *A historical dictionary of psychiatry*. New York: Oxford University Press. ISBN 978-0-19-517668-1. Retrieved 2009-10-01.

[2] Y. A. Adam (March 2007). "Justice in Nuremberg: The Doctors' Trial – 60 Years Later A Reminder" (PDF). *Israel Medical Association Journal* (Israel Medical Association) **9** (3): 194–195. PMID 17402338. Retrieved 2009-10-01.

[3] The Nazi doctors: medical killing and the psychology of genocide pg 122 By Robert Jay Lifton 2000

[4] James M. Glass. "Nuremberg Laws: Genocide and Crimes Against Humanity". eNotes.com, Inc. Retrieved 2009-10-01.

[5] The Strassmanns: Science, Politics and Migration in Turbulent Times (1793-1993)

[6] Remy, Steven P. (2002). *The Heidelberg myth: the Nazification and denazification of a German university*. Cambridge, Massachusetts: Harvard University Press. pp. 118, 138. ISBN 0-674-00933-9. LCCN 2002069072. Retrieved 2009-10-01.

[7] Uwe Henrik Peters, M.D. (2001). "On Nazi Psychiatry" (Fee). *Psychoanalytic Review* (National Psychological Association for Psychoanalysis) **88** (2): 295–309. doi:10.1521/prev.88.2.295.17677. Retrieved 2009-10-01. Schneider also committed suicide, in 1946, while in prison waiting for his trial to begin.

[8] L Singer (December 3, 1998). "Ideology and ethics. The perversion of German psychiatrists' ethics by the ideology of national socialism". *European Psychiatry* (Elsevier SAS) **13** (Supplement 3): 87s–92s. doi:10.1016/S0924-9338(98)80038-2. PMID 19698678. Carl Schneider committed suicide by hanging after his arrest...(subscription required)

21.2 Sources

- Friedlander, Henry (1995). *The Origins of Nazi Genocide: From Euthanasia to the Final Solution*. Chapel

Hill: University of North Carolina Press. ISBN 0-8078-4675-9. Retrieved 2009-10-01.

- Kaplan, Robert M. (2009). *Medical Murder: Disturbing Cases of Doctors Who Kill*. Crows Nest, N.S.W.: Allen & Unwin. ISBN 978-1-74175-610-4. Retrieved 2009-10-01.

- William E. Seidelman (December 7, 1996). "Nuremberg lamentation: for the forgotten victims of medical science". *BMJ* (BMJ Group) **313** (7070): 1463–7. doi:10.1136/bmj.313.7070.1463. PMC 2352986. PMID 8973236.

Chapter 22

Otmar Freiherr von Verschuer

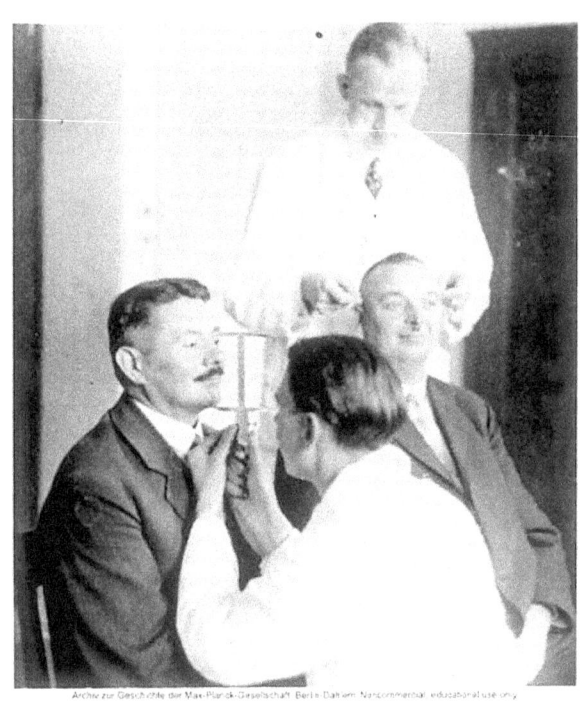

Archiv zur Geschichte der Max-Planck-Gesellschaft, Berlin-Dahlem. Non-commercial, educational use only.

Otmar von Verschuer (rear) supervises the measurement of two men's head circumference as part of an anthropometric study of heredity.

Otmar Freiherr von Verschuer (16 July 1896, Wildeck, Hesse-Nassau – 8 August 1969, Münster, West Germany) was a German human biologist and eugenicist concerned primarily with "racial hygiene" and twin research.[1][2][3] He was the director of the Kaiser Wilhelm Institute of Anthropology, Human Heredity, and Eugenics (*Kaiser-Wilhelm-Institut für Anthropologie, menschliche Erblehre, und Eugenik*; KWIfA) in Berlin and the Institute for Genetic Biology and Racial Hygiene (*Institut für Erbbiologie und Rassenhygiene*).

22.1 Involvement in Nazi human experimentation

He received Heinrich Himmler's permission to work in Auschwitz from 1944 on. One of Verschuer's best known assistants was Josef Mengele, who, as one of the SS physicians at the Auschwitz death camp, later became known as the "Angel of Death".[4]

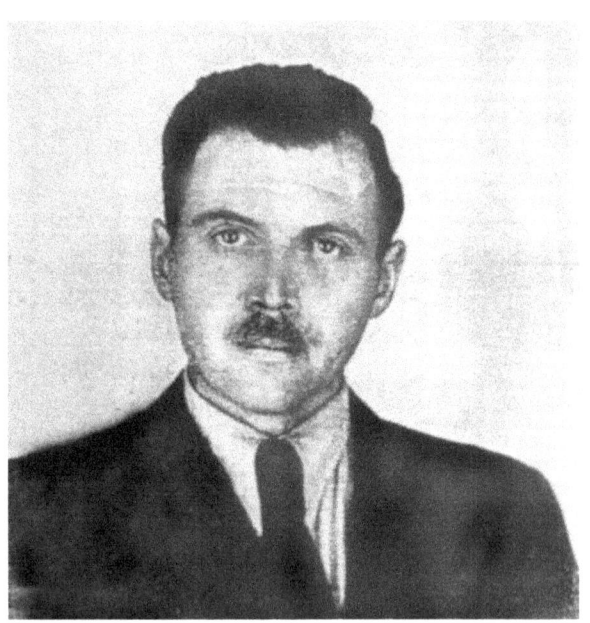

Josef Mengele in 1956. Photo taken by a police photographer in Buenos Aires for Mengele's Argentine identification document.

Verschuer was never tried for war crimes despite many indications that he not only was fully cognisant of Mengele's work at Auschwitz, but even encouraged and collaborated with Mengele in some of his most grisly research. In a report to the German Research Council (*Deutsche Forschungsgemeinschaft*; DFG) from 1944, Verschuer talked about Mengele's assistance in supplying the KWIfA with some "scientific materials" from Auschwitz:

My assistant, Dr. Mengele (M.D., Ph.D.) has joined me in this branch of research. He is presently employed as Hauptsturmführer and camp physician in the concentration camp at Auschwitz. Anthropological investigations on the most diverse racial groups of this concentration camp are being carried out with permission of the SS Reichsführer [Himmler]; the blood samples are being sent to my laboratory for analysis.

Verschuer also noted in the report that the war conditions had made it difficult for the KWIfA to procure "twin materials" for study, and that Mengele's unique position at Auschwitz offered a special opportunity in this respect. In the summer of 1944, Mengele and his Jewish slave assistant Dr. Miklós Nyiszli sent other "scientific materials" to the KWIfA, including the bodies of murdered Gypsies, internal organs of dead children, skeletons of two murdered Jews, and blood samples of twins infected by Mengele with typhus.

22.2   Post-war investigation

However solid evidence of Verschuer's willing collaboration could not be established, much to the disappointment of the principal post-war Allied investigator, Leo Alexander, assigned to his case. In a letter to his wife from 1946, Alexander wrote:

> It sometimes seems as if the Nazis had taken special pains in making practically every nightmare come true. Some new evidence has come in where two doctors in Berlin, one a man and the other a woman, collected eyes of different colour. It seems that the concentration camps were combed for people whose one eye had a slightly different color than the other. Who ever [sic] was unlucky enough to possess such a pair of slightly unequal eyes had them cut out and was killed, the eyes being sent to Berlin. This is the carrying out into reality of an old gruesome German fairy tale, which is included in the Tales of Hoffmann, where Dr Coppelius posing as a sandman comes at night and cuts out children's eyes when they are tired. The grim part of the story is that Doctors von Verschuer and [Karin] Magnussen in Berlin did prefer children and particularly twins. There is no end to this nightmare, at least 23 are being tried now and, I trust, the others will follow later.

Alexander initiated investigations into the location of the incriminating collection but could not locate it—it had been sent to an unknown destination in Berlin and from there vanished out of sight; Alexander ruefully concluded that Verschuer had destroyed it.

Later investigators had difficulty getting hard evidence of the gruesome position they felt Verschuer had in The Holocaust. In his denazification hearing, he was eventually judged as a Nazi fellow traveler (*Mitläufer*) (a relatively mild categorization), fined 600 Reichsmark, and released from custody.

As the war was drawing to a close in 1945, Verschuer moved the files of the KWIfA into the Western part of Germany, hoping for a more favorable response from the advancing Allied armies than from the advancing Soviet Army. In late 1945 or early 1946 he petitioned the mayor of Frankfurt to allow him to reestablish the KWIfA. However the commission in charge of rebuilding the Kaiser Wilhelm Gesellschaft decreed that "Verschuer should be considered not as a collaborator, but one of the most dangerous Nazi activists of the Third Reich." The KWIfA was not reestablished.

In 1951, Verschuer was awarded the prestigious professorship of human genetics at the University of Münster, where he established one of the largest centers of genetics research in West Germany. Like many "racial hygienists" of the Nazi period, and many American eugenicists, Verschuer was successful in redefining himself as a genetics researcher after the war, and avoided the taint of his work with Nazi eugenics. Many of his wartime students were similarly appointed to top positions in universities of Erlangen, Frankfurt, Düsseldorf, and Münster. Karin Magnussen, a biologist whom he worked with, ended up using the eyeballs taken from still-living prisoners at Auschwitz by Dr Josef Mengele for experiments on the pigmentation of the human iris.[5]

He was accepted during the war as a member of the American Eugenics Society, a position he kept until his death.

Verschuer died in 1969 in an automobile accident.

22.3   Partial list of works

- *Erbpathologie* (*Hereditary pathology*,1934).[6]

- *Erbbiologie als Unterlage der Bevölkerungspolitik* (*Hereditary biology as a basis for the population policy*). First published in 1933, re-published and modified in 1936.[6]

- *Rassenhygiene als Wissenschaft und Staatsaufgabe* (*Racial hygiene as Science and State function*, 1936).[6]

- *Leitfaden der Rassenhygiene* (*Textbook of Racial hygiene*, 1944).[6]

- *Eugenik. Kommende Generationen in der Sicht der Genetik* (*Eugenics: Coming Generations in the view of Genetics*, 1966).[6]

22.4   Notes

Regarding personal names: *Freiherr* is a former title (translated as *Baron*), which is now legally a part of the last name. The feminine forms are *Freifrau* and *Freiin*.

[1]   Twin research has been used as a substitute for genetic research and, as such, has been associated with a great deal of scientific fraud; see The "Burt Affair".

[2]   Nicholas Wade, "IQ and Heredity: Suspicion of Fraud Beclouds Classic Experiment", Science 26 November 1976: 916–919.

[3]   D. D. Dorfman, "The Cyril Burt Question: New Findings", Science 29 September 1978: Vol. 201 no. 4362 pp. 1177–1186

[4]   A display of von Verschauer in relation to Mengele appeared during 2011 in the exhibit "Deadly Medicine: Creating the Master Race" in the Museum of Texas Tech University, Lubbock, Texas.Kerns, William (21 February 2011). "Deadly medicine [photo of von Verschuer appears in the print edition only]". *Lubbock Avalanche-Journal*. pp. B1, B4. Retrieved 25 February 2011.

[5]   http://www.dailymail.co.uk/news/article-1142824/Nazi-women-exposed-bit-bad-Hitlers-deranged-male-followers.html

[6]   Westermann, Kühl, Gross (2009), p. 78

22.5   Sources

- Westermann, Stefanie; Kühl, Richard; Gross, Dominik, eds. (2009), Medizin und Nationalsozialismus *vol. 1:* Medizin im Dienst der "Erbgesundheit": Beiträge zur Geschichte der Eugenik und "Rassenhygiene" (*English: Medicine and National Socialism*, Vol. 1: *Medicine at work, the "hereditary health": Contribution to history of Eugenics and "race hygiene"*), LIT Verlag Münster, ISBN 978-3643104786

22.6   See also

- ex-Nazis

- Nazi eugenics

- Dr Heinrich Gross

22.7   References

- Sheila Faith Weiss: *After the Fall. Political Whitewashing, Professional Posturing, and personal Refashioning in the Postwar Career of Otmar Freiherr von Verschuer.* Isis, Vol. 101 (2010), 722–758.

- Peter Degen, "Racial Hygienist Otmar von Verschuer, the Confessing Church, and comparative reflections on postwar rehabilitation," pp. 155–65 in Jing Bao Nie, Japan´s Medical Wartime Atrocities (London: Routledge&Kegan, 2010)

- Robert N. Proctor, *Racial Hygiene: Medicine under the Nazis*, Cambridge, MA: Harvard University Press, 1988.

- Paul Weindling, "'Tales from Nuremberg': The Kaiser Wilhelm Institute for Anthropology and Allied medical war crimes policy," in *Geschichte der Kaiser-Wilhelm-Gesellschaft im Nationalsozialismus: Bestandaufnahme und Perspektiven der Forschung*, ed. Doris Kaufmann, v.2 (Goettingen: Wallstein, 2000), 635–652.

- Katrin Weigmann: "In the name of science. The role of biologists in Nazi atrocities: lessons for today's scientists" in *EMBO Reports* v.2 #10 (2001), 871–875.

- Eric Ehrenreich, "Otmar von Verschuer and the 'Scientific' Legitimization of Nazi Anti-Jewish Policy," *Holocaust and Genocide Studies* 2007 21(1):55–72

22.8   External links

- Works by or about Otmar Freiherr von Verschuer at Internet Archive

- "In the name of science" *EMBO reports* article about KWI scientists' wartime atrocities, with images of Verschuer

- "Skeletons in the Closet of German Science" *Deutsche Welle* article on Verschuer's research connection to Mengele

Chapter 23

Alfred Vierkandt

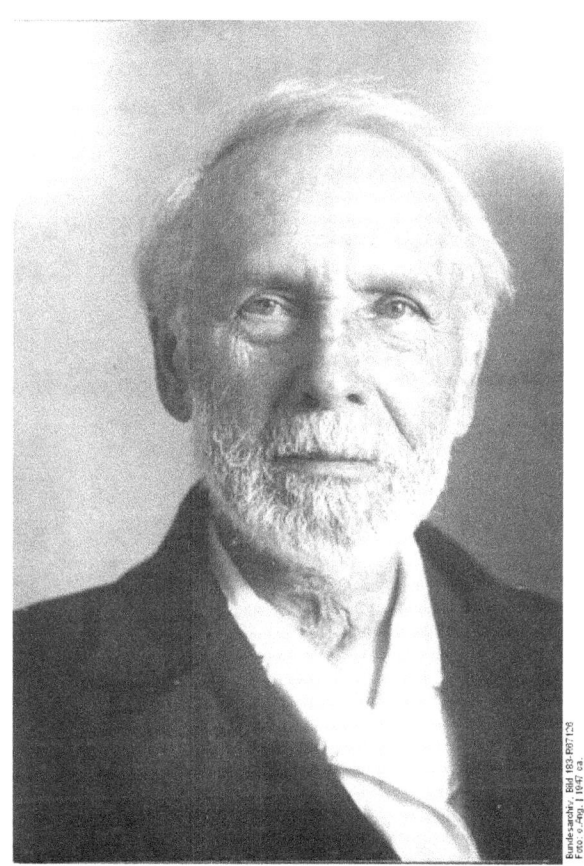

Alfred Vierkandt.

Alfred Vierkandt (4 June 1867 – 24 April 1953) was a German sociologist, ethnographer, social psychologist, social philosopher and philosopher of history. He is known for a broad and phenomenological *Gesellschaftslehre* promulgated in the 1920s, and for his formal sociology.

Vierkandt was born in Hamburg. He first studied science and philosophy at Leipzig University. He habilitated at Brunswick. He was first at *Dozent* in ethnology, becoming eventually in 1913 Professor of Sociology at the University of Berlin. He was one of the founders of the Deutsche Gesellschaft für Soziologie, in 1909. He was made to retire in 1934. He died, aged 85, in Berlin.

23.1 Work

- *Naturvölker und Kulturvölker. Ein Beitrag zur Socialpsychologie* (1896)

- *Die Stetigkeit im Kulturwandel: eine soziologische Studie* (1908)

- *Allgemeine Verfassungs- und Verwaltungsgeschichte* (1911) with Leopold Wenger and others

- *Machtverhältnis und Machtmoral* (1916)

- *Staat und Gesellschaft in der Gegenwart: Eine Einführung in das staatsbürgerliche Denken und in die politische Bewegung unserer Zeit* (1916)

- 'Programm einer formalen Gesellschaftslehre' [Program for a formal theory of society], *Kölner Vierteljahrshefte*, ser. A, Vol. 1, No. 1 (Cologne, 1921)

- *Gesellschaftslehre: Hauptprobleme der philosophischen Soziologie* (1923)

- *Der Dualismus im modernen Weltbild* (1923)

- *Der geistig-sittliche Gehalt des neueren Naturrechtes* (1927)

- *Allgemeine Verfassungs und Verwaltungsgeschichte* (1928)

- *Handwörterbuch der Soziologie* (1931) editor

- *Familie, Volk und Staat in ihren gesellschaftlichen Lebensvorgängen: Eine Einführung in die Gesellschaftslehre* (1936)

- *Kleine Gesellschaftslehre* (1949)

23.2   References

- *Gegenwartsprobleme der Soziologie* (1949) Festschrift

- Paul Hochstim (1966) *Alfred Vierkandt : a sociological critique*

Chapter 24

Werner Villinger

Werner Villinger (9 October 1887 in Besigheim – 8 August 1961 near Innsbruck) was a Nazi German psychiatrist, neurologist, eugenicist and the leading physician at the Bethel Institution ("Anstalt Bethel"). Villinger's specialities included juvenile delinquency, child guidance and group therapy. He was a Professor of Psychiatry at the Philipps University of Marburg and a leading member of the World Federation for Mental Health (WFMH).

Under the Germany's Nazi regime of the 1930s and '40s, Villinger acted as an expert in the government's T-4 Euthanasia Program.

On Social Welfare Education Day 1934, Villinger gave a speech on sterilization and described the reaction, fears and resistance of the boys involved.

He was involved in medical experiments on human beings and ordered thousands to their deaths during the Third Reich but supported Rev. Friedrich von Bodelschwingh's attempt to resist extermination of the mentally ill.

After World War II, Villinger continued his career in the Federal Republic of Germany and co-founded the Federal Ministry of Family, Youth and Health. He was honored by the German government.

Villinger attended the U.S. White House Conference on Children and Youth. In 1951, he became co-chairman of the WFMH Health and Human Relations Conference at Hiddesen-near-Detmold. In 1952, he was a member of a WFMH group on Educating the Public whose Annual Conference met in Brussels. In 1952, he was elected president of the German Association for Child and Youth Psychiatry, and in 1954 became the head of the medical department of Philipps University of Marburg.

In 1961, the German Federal Authorities announced their intent to try Villinger for his actions under the Nazi regime, but before he was brought to trial Villinger threw himself to his death off a mountain top near Innsbruck.

24.1   See also

- Ernst Rüdin

- Euthanasia

- List of Nazi doctors

- Nazi eugenics

24.2   References

- The Origins of Nazi Genocide

- In the Name of the People

- Medical and Psychological Effects of Concentration Camps on Holocaust Survivors

24.3 Text and image sources, contributors, and licenses

24.3.1 Text

- **Wolfgang Abel** *Source:* https://en.wikipedia.org/wiki/Wolfgang_Abel?oldid=687167646 *Contributors:* Graeme Bartlett, Bender235, FlaBot, RussBot, ExRat, Moe Epsilon, Closedmouth, SmackBot, Yannollivier, Iridescent, Goldfritha, Magioladitis, Waacstats, KConWiki, Johnpacklambert, H-Scorpio, Adamdaley, BOTijo, Sitush, Ryleth777, RogDel, Addbot, Lightbot, Yobot, FrescoBot, Full-date unlinking bot, RjwilmsiBot, Bossanoven, Vasstrom, Helpful Pixie Bot, Mazenomda, 14Adrian, ChrisGualtieri, Valleyspring, VIAFbot, KasparBot, TX6785 and Anonymous: 1

- **Otto Ammon** *Source:* https://en.wikipedia.org/wiki/Otto_Ammon?oldid=663401355 *Contributors:* Sheynhertz-Unbayg, Dpv, Intangible, SmackBot, GoodDay, Vina-iwbot~enwiki, Thijs!bot, Waacstats, Lebob, Monegasque, PipepBot, Addbot, Luckas-bot, Erik9bot, DefaultsortBot, Full-date unlinking bot, RjwilmsiBot, Dreambeaver, VIAFbot, KasparBot and Anonymous: 1

- **Gertrud Bäumer** *Source:* https://en.wikipedia.org/wiki/Gertrud_B%C3%A4umer?oldid=678388473 *Contributors:* Bearcat, SlaveToTheWage, Sheynhertz-Unbayg, Stemonitis, RussBot, Intangible, Crystallina, SmackBot, Betacommand, Chicheley, Doug Weller, PetePassword, Nick Number, Waacstats, TXiKiBoT, Logan, Monegasque, Fadesga, RogDel, NobbiP, MystBot, MrR64, Addbot, DOI bot, LaaknorBot, SpBot, Citation bot, نسر برلين, Nightsturm, RjwilmsiBot, Helpful Pixie Bot, Dexbot, VIAFbot, ArmbrustBot, KasparBot and Anonymous: 4

- **Karl Binding** *Source:* https://en.wikipedia.org/wiki/Karl_Binding?oldid=661394175 *Contributors:* Alan Liefting, Jokestress, Ziggurat, Pearle, Dan100, Firsfron, FlaBot, YurikBot, Friedfish, Semperf, Staffelde, Carabinieri, SmackBot, Can't sleep, clown will eat me, Lost in space, Tazmaniacs, Jonathan Groß, Peterlewis, Gondooley, Erik Kennedy, Cydebot, Treybien, Waacstats, R'n'B, Mark v1.0, Broadbot, BOTijo, Mimihitam, Polbot, RogDel, MystBot, Addbot, Zorrobot, Luckas-bot, Neptune5000, Tchussle, Slain34, Green Cardamom, OgreBot, Jonkerz, RjwilmsiBot, FiachraByrne, BG19bot, Ebrequ, VIAFbot, Prokaryotes, KasparBot and Anonymous: 15

- **Agnes Bluhm** *Source:* https://en.wikipedia.org/wiki/Agnes_Bluhm?oldid=696208516 *Contributors:* RussBot, Nikkimaria, Cplakidas, Hebrides, EtienneDolet, Johnpacklambert, Victuallers, Aboutmovies, Yobot, LittleWink, BattyBot, AmericanLemming, KasparBot and Anonymous: 1

- **Hermann Boehm (eugenicist)** *Source:* https://en.wikipedia.org/wiki/Hermann_Boehm_(eugenicist)?oldid=688753895 *Contributors:* Pol098, Lockley, RussBot, Hmains, Neddyseagoon, Cydebot, Magioladitis, Waacstats, Monegasque, Alexander Tendler, Addbot, AnomieBOT, Bossanoven, Aisteco, ÄDA - DÄP and KasparBot

- **Werner Catel** *Source:* https://en.wikipedia.org/wiki/Werner_Catel?oldid=660436376 *Contributors:* HollyAm, Schneelocke, Alan Liefting, WiseWoman, BigBen212, Sherurcij, Nam, SpuriousQ, SmackBot, Intelligent Mr Toad, Lost in space, Bilby, Magioladitis, Waacstats, DGG, R'n'B, Nburden, Java7837, Xdorawinifred, Mimihitam, Good Olfactory, Addbot, TutterMouse, LaaknorBot, Yobot, AnomieBOT, Erik9bot, FrescoBot, RjwilmsiBot, Bossanoven, Bizzurp, VIAFbot, Eustachiusz, KasparBot and Anonymous: 4

- **Eugen Fischer** *Source:* https://en.wikipedia.org/wiki/Eugen_Fischer?oldid=693113175 *Contributors:* Danny, Hephaestos, Paul Barlow, Irmgard, Stone, Ajd, Fastfission, Duncharris, D6, Vsmith, Bender235, MartinSpacek, Woohookitty, Rjwilmsi, Lockley, Olessi, FlaBot, AI, Joonasl, NawlinWiki, Grafen, Vancouveriensis, Shakehandsman, Nikkimaria, Blablabla, SmackBot, Eskimbot, Kintetsubuffalo, Gilliam, John, General Ization, Tazmaniacs, Iglew, Peterlewis, Makyen, OS2Warp, Cydebot, Ward3001, Itsmejudith, Nick Number, PaulVIF, Mengela, Obi-wankenobi, Waacstats, KConWiki, R'n'B, Nono64, Pajfarmor, Alexb102072, Sgeureka, Recato, Moonriddengirl, Monegasque, Ufinne, Sitush, Jrryjude, Staffordshire, Parkwells, Arjayay, Mtsmallwood, Eingangskontrolle, Alexander Tendler, Dthomsen8, Addbot, DOI bot, WikiDreamerBot, Legobot, Yobot, AnomieBOT, MsTingaK, Jim1138, Materialscientist, LilHelpa, Xqbot, Ulf Heinsohn, J04n, GrouchoBot, Omnipaedista, SixBlueFish, FrescoBot, LucienBOT, 3rdWorldkid, Citation bot 1, RedBot, MyMoloboaccount, RjwilmsiBot, Bossanoven, EmausBot, Ferocious osmosis, Italia2006, ZéroBot, Walty1971, Brandmeister, Helpful Pixie Bot, BG19bot, Virago250, Futurist110, VIAFbot, Drtywmn, Prokaryotes, MarkusJPS, Vision2030, KasparBot, Typologist and Anonymous: 35

- **Hermann Gauch** *Source:* https://en.wikipedia.org/wiki/Hermann_Gauch?oldid=689682419 *Contributors:* Paul Barlow, Rjwilmsi, Closedmouth, Betacommand, Cydebot, Epbr123, Waacstats, Thismightbezach, Phil Bridger, Mtsmallwood, Good Olfactory, Mckinley99, SassoBot, Onkel Karlchen, RjwilmsiBot, Bossanoven, Helpful Pixie Bot, BG19bot, ÄDA - DÄP, OccultZone, GingerBreadHarlot, KasparBot and Anonymous: 4

- **Hans F. K. Günther** *Source:* https://en.wikipedia.org/wiki/Hans_F._K._G%C3%BCnther?oldid=695908332 *Contributors:* Paul Barlow, Auric, UtherSRG, Adam McMaster, Klemen Kocjancic, Carptrash, Violetriga, Sleigh, Stemonitis, Kbdank71, JIP, Rjwilmsi, Olessi, Nam, Roboto de Ajvol, RussBot, Maunus, Nikkimaria, Dark Tichondrias, Attilios, SmackBot, Ingsoc, Bluebot, Colonies Chris, Copysan, Will Beback, E-Kartoffel, Cydebot, Tkynerd, Lord of the Isles, Ward3001, Thijs!bot, Olahus, Hmarcuse, JYing, Mengela, J-A-V-A, Xn4, Dienekesp, RoDeWo, Hashomer, Christopherhale, GirasoleDE, Monegasque, Comradesandalio, ImageRemovalBot, PipepBot, Alexbot, PixelBot, TwiLighT1126, MelonBot, Addbot, Luckas-bot, Yobot, Angel ivanov angelov, Omnipaedista, Full-date unlinking bot, Diannaa, Malymac, Bossanoven, EmausBot, WeijiBaikeBianji, Edzard-Freng, Helpful Pixie Bot, Alf.laylah.wa.laylah, Lucy126, VIAFbot, OccultZone, Coat of Many Colours, GingerBreadHarlot, KasparBot, Michael millies and Anonymous: 25

- **Hans Heinze** *Source:* https://en.wikipedia.org/wiki/Hans_Heinze?oldid=662718731 *Contributors:* FeanorStar7, AI, Mark Schierbecker, BG19bot, Eustachiusz, KasparBot and Anonymous: 1

- **Willibald Hentschel** *Source:* https://en.wikipedia.org/wiki/Willibald_Hentschel?oldid=662618883 *Contributors:* Keresaspa, Nikkimaria, Kendrick7, Waacstats, Addbot, RjwilmsiBot, Wbm1058, RobinBnn, JamKaftan, KasparBot and Anonymous: 2

- **Alfred Hoche** *Source:* https://en.wikipedia.org/wiki/Alfred_Hoche?oldid=695168378 *Contributors:* Ugen64, GreatWhiteNortherner, Alan Liefting, Slyguy, TonyW, Kwamikagami, Migozared, Pearle, Rd232, Angr, Rjwilmsi, FlaBot, YurikBot, Tfine80, Epipelagic, Carabinieri, SmackBot, Kintetsubuffalo, Apeloverage, Lost in space, EdGl, Geb11, Peterlewis, Olivierd, CapitalR, Nescio*, Mengela, Gavia immer, Waacstats, Mark v1.0, Monegasque, Mimihitam, Polbot, NuclearWarfare, Addbot, Xqbot, Omnipaedista, Oldfirehall, Green Cardamom, Abductive, DefaultsortBot, RjwilmsiBot, Léon66, ZéroBot, ChuispastonBot, Azooz213, FiachraByrne, Ebrequ, Khazar2, Douglas R. Skopp, VIAFbot, Finnusertop, KasparBot and Anonymous: 17

Trevgreg, Spellmaster, Jonesl84, Cliché guevara, Grimgerde, Smartings, ShaunProm, Cdecoro, PsyMar, MartinBot, SolitaryWolf, RapaNui75, Quickmythril, Rockerdude716, B33R, Timoteostewart, Cooliorobert, RFM57, Nooddawgg, Rettetast, Mitch.sc, InnocuousPseudonym, Birdie, SeeYa32, Bus stop, R'n'B, CommonsDelinker, Nono64, LittleOldMe old, Lilac Soul, Chipdukes, Tgeairn, Dinkytown, RockMFR, J.delanoy, Jahanas, DrKay, Trusilver, Hlnodovic, Parp555, Bogey97, Sp3000, Rsreston, Uncle Dick, STANE, Hodja Nasreddin, Octopus-Hands, Jahredtobin, TomCat4680, EH74DK, Andy5421, Being blunt, Katalaveno, LordAnubisBOT, JayFout, Andrej Kvasnica, Dexter prog, ElectricValkyrie, Congram, AntiSpamBot, ChainSuck-Jimmy, HiLo48, GhostPirate, Alexb102072, Hut 6.5, NewEnglandYankee, Cadwaladr, Taxico, DadaNeem, SJP, Thesis4Eva, Maidenslayer, Macarrones, JHeinonen, T3hllama, Prhartcom, KylieTastic, Barfunkle, Cometstyles, DarkSaber2k, Jimokay, The great rd, Namekal, Dmx100, MishaPan, Ja 62, AndreasJSbot, CA387, Scottydude, Nattfodd, Xiahou, Idioma-bot, Fr33kman, Wikieditor06, Sam Blacketer, Malik Shabazz, Deor, 28bytes, VolkovBot, CWii, Coolman19876545, Zell IW, Himmler14meensmyage, ABF, Viral Slayer, Holme053, Mesmacat, AlnoktaBOT, Gab.popp, Dom Kaos, Toddy1, Philip Trueman, Sağlamcı, Mcjohnz, TXiKiBoT, KevinTR, Vipinhari, CrashingWave, Hayden5650, Rei-bot, Zizibo, Charley sweeney, Doglover2352, Awsemo426, Steven J. Anderson, Cicaneo, Iowamutt, Corvus cornix, SGT141, Gorgon5555, Hoo Hoo Howie!, Familienoriginalbenutzer~enwiki, Josephabradshaw, Jimmybuffet5, Rumiton, Emre43, Pegaroo88, Madhero88, Captaingup, Doug, Gustav Lindwall, Silent52, Plutonium27, TheLoverly, Kittenlvr, Ivanushka~enwiki, Falcon8765, Piratedan, Anna512, Burntsauce, BOTijo, Insanity Incarnate, Northfox, Sarevok1, Krautukie, MetalA, Anickle060193, Chergles, Dusti, OberRanks, OGOL, Caulde, Moonriddengirl, Scarian, Morcus, Schizodelight, Dawn Bard, Karaboom, Wadey4, AFrayMo~enwiki, Quasso, Dinlo juk, BlackSlivers, Mjiadzki, Calabraxthis, Til Eulenspiegel, Oda Mari, Sue Wallace, Monegasque, Strodie, JSpung, Jocedun, Oxymoron83, Jack1956, Antonio Lopez, Harry~enwiki, Steven Crossin, Senor Cuete, Ks0stm, Alex.muller, WacoJacko, Ahangar-e-Gaz, Joaopchagas2, Seventh Ares, JohnSawyer, Spitfire19, Mariaflores1955, MadmanBot, Janggeom, Cyfal, Pinkadelica, Richard David Ramsey, Canglesea, Shlimozzle, Kanonkas, Isthatyoujohnwayneisthisme, Explicit, Steve, RegentsPark, Kobi13, ClueBot, Foxj, The Thing That Should Not Be, All Hallow's Wraith, Rodhullandemu, General Epitaph, Rise Above the Vile, Sierenia, Maru-Spanish, Drmies, Kamix, Pucko67~enwiki, Boing! said Zebedee, OfficeBoy, BANZ111, Otolemur crassicaudatus, Trivialist, Klazno4, Oswego Palomar, Arunsingh16, Puchiko, JustinClarkCasey, Brewcrewer, Dreamspeaker, Excirial, Socrates2008, Jusdafax, Aliasfoxtrot, Jammy0002, John Nevard, Nsmb2, Lartoven, MacedonianBoy, Renzo Grosso, SaneSerenity, Jumanji656, M.O.X, Mtsmallwood, Razorflame, Nicholasweed, 6afraidof7, Polly, Another Believer, John Paul Parks, Thingg, Lindberg, Hellstomper, Aitias, Clippership, Cajunsauce, Versus22, Berean Hunter, Shamanchill, DumZiBoT, Finalnight, InternetMeme, Fastily, Spitfire, Jthughes01, Jdellaro, WillOakland, Doc9871, Shakalooloo Doom, PL290, Truetom, Paragon of Arctic Winter Nights, Mrthomas333, Artaxerxes, Kaiwhakahaere, Rexroad2, Shahinrani, Julystana77, RomanSoldier9001, Ktmrider628, Chasnor15, Addbot, Cheka92, Shaunrobertsmith78, Willking1979, Manuel Trujillo Berges, Some jerk on the Internet, Signthis, Ave Caesar, SnoopleCats, CATMANDOOOOO, Binary TSO, Magus732, VbCrLf, Blethering Scot, Bkmays, Ronhjones, SHarold, PlumCrumbleAndCustard, GD 6041, Menne12345, CanadianLinuxUser, Fluffernutter, Zanzibar666, Ka Faraq Gatri, Orange Carrot, Benjomania, Ebaumsworlddotcom001, Download, Glane23, Debresser, SteveLaino, Favonian, Setwisohi, Theking17825, Tide rolls, Luckas Blade, Marksdaman, Ben Ben, Legobot, Luckas-bot, Yobot, Discourseur, Fraggle81, Donfbreed, Evans1982, The Earwig, Reenem, Matanya, Mr T (Based), Hadding, IW.HG, BeBoldInEdits, Magog the Ogre, Anonymous from the 21th century, AnomieBOT, Mike Hayes, Hairhorn, Peril, Crecy99, RandomAct, Materialscientist, Eeems, E2eamon, Eumolpo, Keystoneridin, Clark89, Quebec99, Gsmgm, FreeRangeFrog, Xqbot, Zad68, Sionus, St.nerol, Alexlange, Capricorn42, Baseballjarrett, Weathergirl123, Jsharpminor, Tyrol5, Srich32977, WotWeiller, Vasant56, Horroroftheteenagelobstercello, J04n, C+C, REVUpminster, Alumnum, Omnipaedista, Anotherclown, Mvaldemar, NOLA504ever, Zeldakitten, Doulos Christos, Zzzlugnut, Gtamob69, Thatdoodwithglasses, Pelirrojo778, E0steven, ⁇, X-ponerd20, Erik9, Mjasfca, ProfessorThompson, Green Cardamom, Dan6hell66, Hemuln, Accretianboy, FrescoBot, Facefartmaster, NAKALAK, Surv1v4l1st, Kierzek, Tobby72, Rrrick333, Tobetheman, KMFDM Fan, Super soaker15, HJ Mitchell, CHARGERLEVANI, Ghouse78, Weetoddid, Pxos, Citation bot 1, RaveDog, DrilBot, Alonso de Mendoza, Tinton5, Wikitanvir, VenomousConcept, Cramyourspam, NFSreloaded, Wusha, Vrenator, Thesniperremix, Dcs002, Cassianto, Reaper Eternal, Ktlynch, Diannaa, ThinkEnemies, Tbhotch, Stianh22, DARTH SIDIOUS 2, RjwilmsiBot, Bento00, Bossanoven, Beyond My Ken, Polylepsis, Immunize, Dadaist6174, Nerissa-Marie, GoingBatty, Smitty1337, Bt8257, Tommy2010, TEHodson, Wikipelli, Mikemacdee, BurtAlert, Cogiati, Illegitimate Barrister, Bongoramsey, Fæ, Josve05a, Countess of Landsfield, ElationAviation, Anir1uph, AOC25, Dunblas, Davisdigi, Laelius Linguae, Drcjel, IcehouseCover, Ikemanfow, Wingman4l7, Jonathan Snack, Gratkkk, Usb10, Ego White Tray, Mystichumwipe, Razzattack, Mcc1789, AxMan11, 19thPharaoh, Brutal Adept, Winnipeger16, ClueBot NG, Serasuna, FourLights, WPWWHH1488, Jkta97, Slartibartfastibast, Crassybassy, Joetlawrence2004, Goochgooch, Widr, PaoloNapolitano, Pudge MclameO, LucasNHall, Jjmax5, StrawberryGURL, Helpful Pixie Bot, Atenstaedt, Newyork1501, LiLKingDog, Calabe1992, Jackdawson1970, Hengist Pod, Lowercase sigmabot, BG19bot, Arnavchaudhary, MariceEttlinCaro, Meepiemcmeep, Julien16, Msaunier, Neil Gibbons, MusikAnimal, Kendall-K1, Badon, AwamerT, Virago250, Piguy101, InvestigativeReporter, J R Gainey, Lolo7890, Slushy9, Jorgealamilla, Glacialfox, Hoiguy, Loudmoner, Masonfreemason, Echolima47, Trishawiki, Alexandra Golda, Vanished user lt94ma34le12, Fraulein451, Jimw338, Calebgeske, Mediran, Tandrum, Bardrick, Ekren, Lindsla, ÄDA - DÄP, Dexbot, Mogism, DJ-Joker16, Cuddyc, UselessToRemain, Dirk Küchmeister, Edmond Honda, VIAFbot, Zakr07, 93, Silverback2173, BrokenArticlesLOL, Isaacshackleford, BirgittaMTh, Beppo911, Epicgenius, Mr. Watson (before the phd), Figfoe89, Marchino61, Comp.arch, Prokaryotes, Pietro13, Hitcher vs. Candyman, Jonas Vinther, Marcest19xx, MCarsten, Elmeanopeno, Filedelinkerbot, Signthis1, Gfdsasd, Lizzles86, TridiaChaplain, Youngdrake, Peralta2305, Cirflow, Lux ex Tenebris, KasparBot, TX6785 and Anonymous: 1507

- **Otfrid Mittmann** *Source:* https://en.wikipedia.org/wiki/Otfrid_Mittmann?oldid=652972549 *Contributors:* Waacstats, Wgolf, Jochen Burghardt and EoRdE6

- **Alfred Ploetz** *Source:* https://en.wikipedia.org/wiki/Alfred_Ploetz?oldid=698950487 *Contributors:* Paul Barlow, Irmgard, Samsara, Rich Farmbrough, Bender235, Pearle, Abanima, Richard Arthur Norton (1958-), Kelisi, GregorB, Lockley, AI, Str1977, Jaraalbe, Volunteer Marek, Carabinieri, Ketil3, Crystallina, SmackBot, Richfife, Miquonranger03, CmdrObot, KarlV, Cydebot, Doug Weller, I like Burke's Peerage, Mrund, Waacstats, Ncondee, Victuallers, VolkovBot, Hartmut Haberland, Northfox, Monegasque, All Hallow's Wraith, Addbot, Luckas-bot, Angel ivanov angelov, Hadding, Materialscientist, Irredeemableblogger, Green Cardamom, Lotje, RjwilmsiBot, Bossanoven, Léon66, AvicAWB, Helpful Pixie Bot, BattyBot, VIAFbot, Prokaryotes, Wishfulness, KasparBot, Belovaci and Anonymous: 20

- **Ernst Rüdin** *Source:* https://en.wikipedia.org/wiki/Ernst_R%C3%BCdin?oldid=694724924 *Contributors:* Deb, Paul Barlow, Irmgard, Stone, Stewartadcock, Duncharris, DNewhall, Klemen Kocjancic, D6, Rich Farmbrough, Bender235, Christian Kreibich, Pearle, Gene Nygaard, AI, Gparker, Maustrauser, Bgwhite, UkPaolo, Wavelength, RussBot, Gardar Rurak, THB, Maunus, Tilman, NeilN, Blablabla, Attilios, SmackBot, Hmains, GoodDay, ArglebargleIV, DavidCooke, Lapaz, Jetman, Cydebot, Doug Weller, CopperKettle, Mengela, List of marijuana slang terms, Waacstats, Grandia01, R'n'B, VolkovBot, Oshwah, Mark v1.0, ^demonBot2, PolarBot, ImageRemovalBot, All Hallow's Wraith, Cirt, Gennarous, Addbot, DOI bot, Lightbot, RobSchop, AnomieBOT, FrescoBot, Citation bot 1, Full-date unlinking bot, Wuermler, RjwilmsiBot, John of

Reading, Hydrocarbonic, Kugao, ClueBot NG, FiachraByrne, ÄDA - DÄP, VIAFbot, Monkbot, Wishfulness, KasparBot and Anonymous: 22

- **Carl Schneider** *Source:* https://en.wikipedia.org/wiki/Carl_Schneider?oldid=698680217 *Contributors:* Bearcat, Rjwilmsi, Bgwhite, Anders.Warga, GoodDay, Cydebot, EverSince, S. M. Sullivan, MystBot, Addbot, Luckas-bot, Yobot, Omnipaedista, Citation bot 1, RjwilmsiBot, Bossanoven, Hydrocarbonic, AManWithNoPlan, ClueBot NG, FiachraByrne, Helpful Pixie Bot, VIAFbot, Stamptrader, Monkbot, Wishfulness, KasparBot and Anonymous: 3

- **Otmar Freiherr von Verschuer** *Source:* https://en.wikipedia.org/wiki/Otmar_Freiherr_von_Verschuer?oldid=663536619 *Contributors:* Schneelocke, Dimadick, Fastfission, Duncharris, DO'Neil, Roisterer, Jokestress, StanZegel, MarkusHagenlocher, SteveCrook, Gryffindor, Lockley, Olessi, AI, Rbonvall, YurikBot, Retaggio, PhilipC, Maunus, Deville, Bayerischermann, SmackBot, Colonies Chris, PieRRoMaN, Ohconfucius, Ser Amantio di Nicolao, Tazmaniacs, Cydebot, Itsmejudith, Mengela, HanzoHattori, Wasell, Katalaveno, Mark v1.0, Moonriddengirl, Monegasque, Richard David Ramsey, Sitush, Ejehrenr, ClueBot, Addbot, Green Squares, Lightbot, Zorrobot, Yobot, 2D, Darolew, J04n, Omnipaedista, Groq5, Green Cardamom, Chenopodiaceous, RjwilmsiBot, Bossanoven, Virago250, Fylbecatulous, Sequoia7, ÄDA - DÄP, VIAFbot, OccultZone, Lizzles86, KasparBot and Anonymous: 33

- **Alfred Vierkandt** *Source:* https://en.wikipedia.org/wiki/Alfred_Vierkandt?oldid=686180928 *Contributors:* Magnus Manske, Deb, Charles Matthews, Topbanana, YurikBot, Intangible, Neier, SmackBot, Ser Amantio di Nicolao, Cydebot, Travelbird, Waacstats, Johnpacklambert, BOTijo, Le Pied-bot~enwiki, Zxly, Addbot, Raven1977, Full-date unlinking bot, RjwilmsiBot, Alexpostfacto, VIAFbot, KasparBot and Anonymous: 2

- **Werner Villinger** *Source:* https://en.wikipedia.org/wiki/Werner_Villinger?oldid=670073755 *Contributors:* Edward, Irmgard, Rebrane, Darwinek, Pearle, Kbdank71, Exeunt, AI, BirgitteSB, SmackBot, Robth, DavidCooke, Keith-264, Cydebot, AniMate, Jammy simpson, Otto4711, Mengela, Nono64, Mark v1.0, BOTijo, Rjd0060, Straightway, Mtsmallwood, Gennarous, Addbot, Magus732, LaaknorBot, Debresser, Lightbot, SoiledDishcloth, Pflastertreter, RjwilmsiBot, Bossanoven, Furor Teutonicus, Decathlete, VIAFbot, OccultZone, KasparBot and Anonymous: 2

24.3.2 Images

- **File:66935A.jpeg** *Source:* https://upload.wikimedia.org/wikipedia/commons/5/51/Child_survivors_of_Auschwitz.jpeg *License:* Public domain *Contributors:* USHMM/Belarusian State Archive of Documentary Film and Photography http://collections.ushmm.org/search/catalog/pa14532 *Original artist:* Alexander Voronzow and others in his group, ordered by Mikhael Oschurkow, head of the photography unit

- **File:Alfred_Erich_Hoche.jpg** *Source:* https://upload.wikimedia.org/wikipedia/commons/4/46/Alfred_Erich_Hoche.jpg *License:* Public domain *Contributors:* Die Medizin der Gegenwart in Selbstdarstellungen , Grote LR, editor. Leipzig: Verlag von Felix Meiner, 1923 Frontispice retrieved from: Falzeder EM, Burnham JC. A perfectly staged 'concerted action' against psychoanalysis. The International Journal of Psychoanalysis. 2007 Oct;88(5):1223-1244 *Original artist:* anonymous/unknown

- **File:Alfred_Ploetz.jpg** *Source:* https://upload.wikimedia.org/wikipedia/commons/4/4a/Alfred_Ploetz.jpg *License:* Public domain *Contributors:* http://ihm.nlm.nih.gov/images/B20865 *Original artist:* J.F. Lehmann (1864-1935), Munich, Galerie Hervorr.

- **File:Bundesarchiv_Bild_183-1989-0912-500,_Prof._Hans_Günther.jpg** *Source:* https://upload.wikimedia.org/wikipedia/commons/6/6c/Bundesarchiv_Bild_183-1989-0912-500%2C_Prof._Hans_G%C3%BCnther.jpg *License:* CC BY-SA 3.0 de *Contributors:* This image was provided to Wikimedia Commons by the German Federal Archive (Deutsches Bundesarchiv) as part of a cooperation project. The German Federal Archive guarantees an authentic representation only using the originals (negative and/or positive), resp. the digitalization of the originals as provided by the Digital Image Archive. *Original artist:* Unknown

- **File:Bundesarchiv_Bild_183-1998-0817-502,_Berlin,_Kundgebung_an_der_Universität.jpg** *Source:* https://upload.wikimedia.org/wikipedia/commons/6/65/Bundesarchiv_Bild_183-1998-0817-502%2C_Berlin%2C_Kundgebung_an_der_Universit%C3%A4t.jpg *License:* CC BY-SA 3.0 de *Contributors:* This image was provided to Wikimedia Commons by the German Federal Archive (Deutsches Bundesarchiv) as part of a cooperation project. The German Federal Archive guarantees an authentic representation only using the originals (negative and/or positive), resp. the digitalization of the originals as provided by the Digital Image Archive. *Original artist:* Unknown

- **File:Bundesarchiv_Bild_183-R67126,_Alfred_Vierkandt.jpg** *Source:* https://upload.wikimedia.org/wikipedia/commons/7/70/Bundesarchiv_Bild_183-R67126%2C_Alfred_Vierkandt.jpg *License:* CC BY-SA 3.0 de *Contributors:* This image was provided to Wikimedia Commons by the German Federal Archive (Deutsches Bundesarchiv) as part of a cooperation project. The German Federal Archive guarantees an authentic representation only using the originals (negative and/or positive), resp. the digitalization of the originals as provided by the Digital Image Archive. *Original artist:* Unknown

- **File:Bundesarchiv_Bild_183-S72707,_Heinrich_Himmler.jpg** *Source:* https://upload.wikimedia.org/wikipedia/commons/7/79/Bundesarchiv_Bild_183-S72707%2C_Heinrich_Himmler.jpg *License:* CC BY-SA 3.0 de *Contributors:* This image was provided to Wikimedia Commons by the German Federal Archive (Deutsches Bundesarchiv) as part of a cooperation project. The German Federal Archive guarantees an authentic representation only using the originals (negative and/or positive), resp. the digitalization of the originals as provided by the Digital Image Archive. *Original artist:* Friedrich Franz Bauer

- **File:Commons-logo.svg** *Source:* https://upload.wikimedia.org/wikipedia/en/4/4a/Commons-logo.svg *License:* ? *Contributors:* ? *Original artist:* ?

- **File:Crystal_personal.svg** *Source:* https://upload.wikimedia.org/wikipedia/en/2/24/Crystal_personal.svg *License:* ? *Contributors:* ? *Original artist:* ?

- **File:DBP_1974_793_Gertrud_Bäumer.jpg** *Source:* https://upload.wikimedia.org/wikipedia/commons/a/a0/DBP_1974_793_Gertrud_B%C3%A4umer.jpg *License:* Public domain *Contributors:* scanned by NobbiP *Original artist:* scanned by NobbiP

- **File:Esclapius_stick.svg** *Source:* https://upload.wikimedia.org/wikipedia/commons/7/7a/Esclapius_stick.svg *License:* Public domain *Contributors:* No machine-readable source provided. Own work assumed (based on copyright claims). *Original artist:* No machine-readable author provided. Melian assumed (based on copyright claims).

- **File:Eugen_Fischer.jpg** *Source:* https://upload.wikimedia.org/wikipedia/en/0/0d/Eugen_Fischer.jpg *License:* Fair use *Contributors:* http://www.eugenicsarchive.org *Original artist:* ?

- **File:Flag_Schutzstaffel.svg** *Source:* https://upload.wikimedia.org/wikipedia/commons/3/33/Flag_Schutzstaffel.svg *License:* Public domain *Contributors:* Flag Schutzstaffel.gif: <a href='//commons.wikimedia.org/wiki/File:Flag_Schutzstaffel.gif' class='image'><img alt='Flag Schutzstaffel.gif' src='https://upload.wikimedia.org/wikipedia/commons/thumb/1/1c/Flag_Schutzstaffel.gif/18px-Flag_Schutzstaffel.gif' width='18' height='12' srcset='https://upload.wikimedia.org/wikipedia/commons/thumb/1/1c/Flag_Schutzstaffel.gif/27px-Flag_Schutzstaffel. gif 1.5x, https://upload.wikimedia.org/wikipedia/commons/thumb/1/1c/Flag_Schutzstaffel.gif/36px-Flag_Schutzstaffel.gif 2x' data-file- width='324' data-file-height='216' /></a> *Original artist:* NielsF

- **File:Flag_of_Bavaria_(lozengy).svg** *Source:* https://upload.wikimedia.org/wikipedia/commons/2/20/Flag_of_Bavaria_%28lozengy%29.svg *License:* Public domain *Contributors:*

- Bundeszentrale für politische Bildung: *Wappen und Flaggen der Bundesrepublik Deutschland und ihrer Länder* 3. Auflage. Magdeburger Druckerei GmbH, Bonn 1994, ISBN 3-89331-206-4. *Original artist:* diese Datei: Jwnabd

- **File:Flag_of_German_Reich_(1935–1945).svg** *Source:* https://upload.wikimedia.org/wikipedia/commons/9/99/Flag_of_German_Reich_ %281935%E2%80%931945%29.svg *License:* Public domain *Contributors:* Own work *Original artist:* Fornax

- **File:Flag_of_Germany.svg** *Source:* https://upload.wikimedia.org/wikipedia/en/b/ba/Flag_of_Germany.svg *License:* PD *Contributors:* ? *Original artist:* ?

- **File:Flag_of_the_German_Empire.svg** *Source:* https://upload.wikimedia.org/wikipedia/commons/e/ec/Flag_of_the_German_Empire.svg *License:* Public domain *Contributors:* Recoloured Image:Flag of Germany (2-3).svg *Original artist:* User:B1mbo and User:Madden

- **File:Flag_of_the_NSDAP_(1920–1945).svg** *Source:* https://upload.wikimedia.org/wikipedia/commons/c/cf/Flag_of_the_NSDAP_ %281920%E2%80%931945%29.svg *License:* Public domain *Contributors:* Original PNG version created by de:Benutzer:Kookaburra with the name "Bild:Flag Germany 1933.png" in de.wikipedia; uploaded to the Wikimedia Commons by User:Guanaco, later converted to SVG by User:Rotemliss and later modified by other Wikimedia Commons people. *Original artist:* ?

- **File:Gedenktafel_Alt-Reinickendorf_45_(Reini)_Max_Julius_Hodann.JPG** *Source:* https://upload.wikimedia.org/wikipedia/commons/ 7/7f/Gedenktafel_Alt-Reinickendorf_45_%28Reini%29_Max_Julius_Hodann.JPG *License:* CC BY-SA 3.0 *Contributors:* Own work *Original artist:* OTFW, Berlin

- **File:Hans_F._K._Günther_-_Short_Ethnology_of_the_German_People_(1929)_pp._34-5.jpg** *Source:* https://upload.wikimedia.org/ wikipedia/en/a/ab/Hans_F._K._G%C3%BCnther_-_Short_Ethnology_of_the_German_People_%281929%29_pp._34-5.jpg *License:* Fair use *Contributors:* https://archive.org/details/Guenther-Hans-Kleine-Rassenkunde-des-deutschen-Volkes-Text *Original artist:* Hans F. K. Günther

- **File:Hermann_Boehm_at_the_Nuremberg_Trials.jpg** *Source:* https://upload.wikimedia.org/wikipedia/commons/c/cc/Hermann_Boehm_ at_the_Nuremberg_Trials.jpg *License:* Public domain *Contributors:* http://forum.axishistory.com/download/file.php?id=104457 *Original artist:* US Army photographers on behalf of the OCCWC

- **File:Jane_Goodall_HK.jpg** *Source:* https://upload.wikimedia.org/wikipedia/commons/d/dc/Jane_Goodall_HK.jpg *License:* CC BY 2.5 *Contributors:* Self-published work by Jeekc *Original artist:* Jeekc

- **File:Josef_Mengele.jpg** *Source:* https://upload.wikimedia.org/wikipedia/en/f/fc/Josef_Mengele.jpg *License:* Fair use *Contributors:* http://www.timetoast.com/timelines/josef-mengele *Original artist:* ?

- **File:Josef_Mengele_Signature.svg** *Source:* https://upload.wikimedia.org/wikipedia/commons/e/e2/Josef_Mengele_Signature.svg *License:* Public domain *Contributors:* Traced in Adobe Illustrator from http://www.museumofworldwarii.com/Images2005/07mengelelg.gif *Original artist:* Josef Mengele

- **File:Karl_Binding.jpeg** *Source:* https://upload.wikimedia.org/wikipedia/commons/8/80/Karl_Binding.jpeg *License:* Public domain *Contributors:* de.wikipedia; transferred to Commons by User:Kelly using CommonsHelper. (Original text : *Vor dem 1. Januar 1923 veröffentlicht*) *Original artist:* Unknown; original uploader was Matthias Bock at de.wikipedia

- **File:NewtonDetail.jpg** *Source:* https://upload.wikimedia.org/wikipedia/commons/3/35/NewtonDetail.jpg *License:* Public domain *Contributors:* Transferred from en.wikipedia to Commons by Sreejithk2000 using CommonsHelper. *Original artist:* The original uploader was Trovatore at English Wikipedia

- **File:Question_book-new.svg** *Source:* https://upload.wikimedia.org/wikipedia/en/9/99/Question_book-new.svg *License:* Cc-by-sa-3.0 *Contributors:*
  Created from scratch in Adobe Illustrator. Based on Image:Question book.png created by User:Equazcion *Original artist:*
  Tkgd2007

- **File:SS-Hauptsturmführer_Collar_Rank.svg** *Source:* https://upload.wikimedia.org/wikipedia/commons/4/4b/SS-Hauptsturmf%C3% BChrer_Collar_Rank.svg *License:* CC BY-SA 3.0 *Contributors:* Own work *Original artist:* Mintz l

- **File:SS-Untersturmführer_Collar_Rank.svg** *Source:* https://upload.wikimedia.org/wikipedia/commons/a/a7/SS-Untersturmf%C3% BChrer_Collar_Rank.svg *License:* CC BY-SA 3.0 *Contributors:* Own work *Original artist:* Mintz l

- **File:Scientist.svg** *Source:* https://upload.wikimedia.org/wikipedia/commons/0/03/Scientist.svg *License:* CC-BY-SA-3.0 *Contributors:* Own work *Original artist:* Viktorvoigt

- **File:Selection_Birkenau_ramp.jpg** *Source:* https://upload.wikimedia.org/wikipedia/commons/8/89/Selection_Birkenau_ramp.jpg *License:* Public domain *Contributors:* Yad Vashem. The album was donated to Yad Vashem by Lili Jacob, a survivor, who found it in the Mittelbau-Dora concentration camp in 1945. *Original artist:* Unknown. Several sources believe the photographer to have been Ernst Hoffmann or Bernhard Walter of the SS

24.3.3 Content license